foods
to fight
cancer

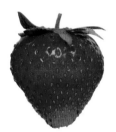

cabbage

raspberries

turmeric

garlic

wine

blueberries

onion

orange

tomato

foods
to fight
cancer

Essential foods to help
prevent cancer

Richard Béliveau, Ph.d.
Denis Gingras, Ph.d.

LONDON, NEW YORK,
MELBOURNE, MUNICH, and DELHI

Project Editor Kathy Fahey
Project Designer Jo Grey
Senior Editor Jennifer Latham
Senior Art Editor Peggy Sadler
Managing Editor Penny Warren
Managing Art Editor Marianne Markham
Publishing Director Mary-Clare Jerram
DTP Designer Sonia Charbonnier
Production Controller Stuart Masheter
Jacket Designer Neal Cobourne

First American Edition, 2007

Published in the United States by
DK Publishing
375 Hudson Street
New York, New York 10014

08 09 10 11   10 9 8 7 6 5 4 3 2
FD136–May 2007

Published in Great Britain by
Dorling Kindersley Limited.

A catalog record for this book is available
from the Library of Congress

ISBN 978-0-7566-2867-3

Color reproduction by GRB
Printed and bound in Hong Kong by
Sheck Wah Tong

Discover more at
www.dk.com

Contents

Part one
Cancer, A Formidable Enemy

Part two
Nutraceuticals: Foods That Fight Cancer

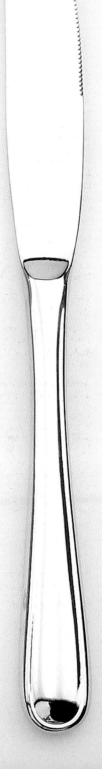

Part three
Day-to-day Nutrition
Therapy

Preface by Pierre Bruneau

This book is essential reading for all those who have taken an interest in cancer. Essential, because it gives us the opportunity, perhaps for the first time, to understand the perspective of scientists who are actively involved in the field of cancer research, to measure exactly how much progress has been made and, even more importantly, to learn about the means now at our disposal to fight this terrible disease. Although we are now overwhelmed by an incredible amount of contradictory information about cancer, this book offers the general public a wealth of straightforward facts that will enable you to make sense of the current data.

Whether or not we and our loved ones have personally been touched by cancer, we must admit that this disease has the power to trouble us... What, if anything, can be done to prevent it? And if our lives are touched by cancer, as mine was, we tell ourselves that "everything" must be tried in an attempt to cure the disease. I lived through this experience with my son Charles... At the beginning of his illness, we asked ourselves if there was anything we could have done, or anything more we could do!

Much more than a popular science treatise, this book proposes a profound and far-reaching reflection on the impact that our lifestyle choices, particularly the ones that predominate in industrialized nations today, may have on the risks of being afflicted by cancer. In this time of technological prowess without precedent, when we put all our hopes and considerable energies in the discovery of medicines designed to cure cancer, have we really thought about what we might do to prevent its appearance? Could the ever-growing number of certain cancers observed in recent years be related to important changes that have occurred in the way we live? Are we really using all available resources to fight this disease? In my opinion, this book provides a major contribution to our perception of cancer: fighting cancer means not only conquering the tumors that have already manifested themselves in our bodies, but also doing everything possible so that smaller tumors do not get a chance to develop.

We often hear specialists emphasize the importance of eating a balanced diet in order to remain fit and healthy; this book goes much further, by showing how everyday, humble-seeming foods – cabbage, for instance, or garlic, or our delicious summer berries – contain extremely powerful molecules that fight cancer by acting at the very source of the disease: by fighting its development. Eating is not an act devoid of consequences; in fact, the very opposite is true. It is without a doubt the simplest, most basic and natural way to actively arm oneself against a foe as formidable as cancer.

This extraordinary, magnificently illustrated book combines the scientific rigor of its primary argument with anecdotes from history and literature, and even some poetry, while remaining a concise and practical guide. I am convinced that it will change forever your perception of cancer and of the actions we need to take to conquer this disease.

PIERRE BRUNEAU
Journalist

Preface by William W. Li

Food is one the essentials of human existence, with its selection, combination, and transformation a privilege enjoyed exclusively by Man. Ancient cultures developed traditions recognizing the intrinsic, healthful properties of food ingredients, including vegetables, fruits, legumes, and spices – and incorporating them into daily living with wellness in mind. Ironically, modern medicine offers a reverse perspective on food. Patients receive dietary advice from physicians usually only after disease is entrenched in the body. The advice given is almost always negative: avoid this, eliminate that, no fats, no sugars, no meats, no alcohol, no caffeine, and so on. Most medical doctors, in fact, are neither educated nor knowledgeable about the scientific basis behind health-promoting factors found in the diet.

Yet patients and the public crave this information, and devour information on antioxidants, phytochemicals, and other substances present in food. In this timely and beautiful book, Drs Béliveau and Gingras, both internationally renowned cancer researchers, bring forth the cutting-edge scientific facts about diet in a remarkable, easy to understand way designed for all audiences. They authoritatively discuss the history behind foods, spices, beverages such as green tea, turmeric, berries, and even chocolate, taking the reader on a journey from the past to the scientific present of dietary knowledge. Their focus is on cancer, and their discussion includes suggestions on how

dietary factors may be rationally incorporated in daily living with the goals of cancer prevention and disease suppression. The authors combine their decades of scientific research experience to explain how genetic and cellular forces conspire to cause cancer and enable its spread throughout the body as metastases. Then, they describe how substances naturally present in foods possess the biochemical ability to prevent, thwart, and reverse cancer-promoting mechanisms in the body. In particular, this book is the first to discuss how tumor angiogenesis, the growth of new blood vessels that feed cancer cells, may be inhibited by dietary factors. Dr. Béliveau's laboratory in Montreal has pioneered modern methods to study the links between diet and angiogenesis in a systematic and comprehensive fashion – and Dr. Béliveau himself is truly one of the visionary innovators of the new science of food. While biotechnology companies are busy creating designer drugs to conquer cancer, readers of this book will learn new concepts on how dietary choices may influence and suppress tumor development. As 21st-century medicine unravels the mysteries of disease, some of the answers to cancer may indeed lie in our diet.

Foods to Fight Cancer is superbly illustrated and written by two of the world's most innovative scientists today – offering readers a perspective and prescription to health that may be obtained not in the hospital and pharmacy, but in the market and kitchen.

WILLIAM W. LI, M.D.
President and Medical Director, The Angiogenesis Foundation
Cambridge, Massachusetts, USA

Foreword

Cancer continues to defy the progress made by modern medicine; after over forty years of intensive research, it remains a mysterious killer, responsible for the premature deaths of millions of people each year. If certain cancers are now treated with a good degree of success, many others are still very difficult to fight and represent a major cause of mortality among the active population. Now, more than ever, discovering new means of increasing the effectiveness of current anticancer therapies is of great importance.

The goal of this book is to present a summary of the scientific studies currently available. These studies strongly suggest that certain types of cancer can be prevented by modifying our dietary habits to include foods with the power to fight tumors at the source and thus prevent their growth. Nature supplies us with an abundance of foods rich in molecules with very powerful anticancer properties, capable of engaging with the disease without causing any harmful side effects. In many respects, these foods possess therapeutic properties on a par with those of synthetic drugs; we propose calling them "nutraceuticals" to better illustrate these properties. We have the possibility of deploying a veritable arsenal of anticancer compounds occurring naturally in many foods as a complement to the therapies now in use. We can seize this occasion to change the probabilities in our favor, since a diet based on a regular intake of nutraceuticals may indeed prevent the appearance of many different types of cancer.

RICHARD BÉLIVEAU AND DENIS GINGRAS

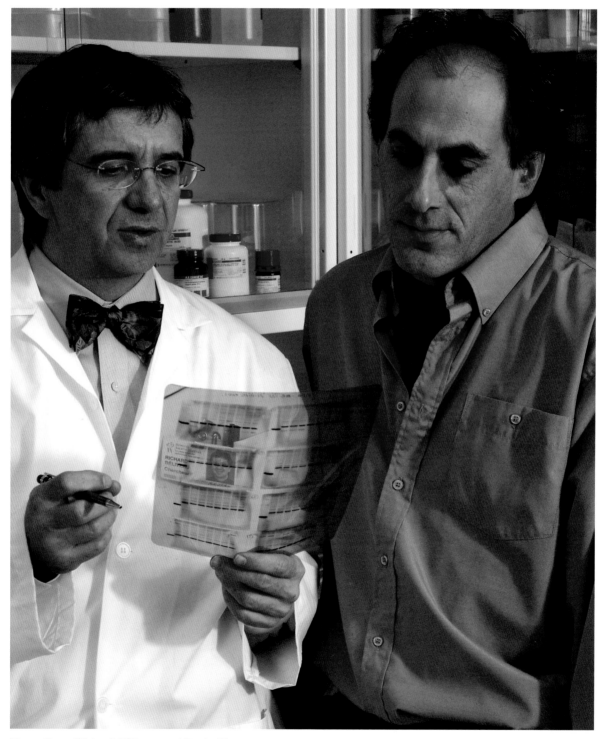

The authors Richard Béliveau and Denis Gingras

part 1

Cancer
a formidable enemy

- The Curse of Cancer

- What is Cancer?

- Preventing Cancer Growth

- Eating to Prevent Cancer

- Phytochemicals and Health

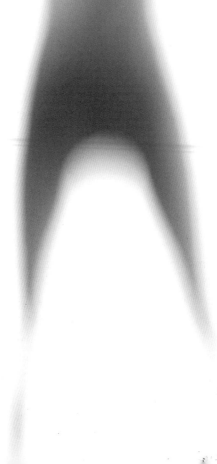

"Almost all of life's misfortunes come from false ideas we hold about what is happening to us."

Stendhal, *Journal* (1801–1805)

The Curse
of Cancer

Most people fear cancer but also believe that there is little they can do to prevent it. They put developing cancer down to hereditary factors or sheer bad luck. However, scientific research shows that this is not the case, and that lifestyle factors such as diet can play a major role in preventing cancer.

THE STATISTICS OF CANCER

Some people have an irrational fear of flying; others are terrified by the idea of sharks or lightning: fearing fatal consequences that might arise from events beyond our control is, after all, a very human characteristic. Yet the real risks of such catastrophes are relatively minor compared to risks directly associated with daily life (**see Figure 1, p.14**). For example, people who are obese have a risk of dying prematurely of causes linked to their excess weight that is almost one million times greater than that of being in an airplane crash; any one of us is at least 50,000 times more likely to be struck by cancer than by lightning over the course of our lifetime, and this risk is even greater if we engage in high-risk behavior such as smoking. Among the dangers that we all have to face at some point in our

lives, cancer presents a very real threat: it will affect one person in three before the age of 75, and one person in four will die from complications caused by the disease. Every year, ten million people in the world develop cancer and seven million deaths are caused by the disease; this corresponds to 12 percent of all reported deaths on Earth. And the world-wide situation is not getting any rosier, since it is now estimated that with the progressive aging of the population, over fifteen million new cases will be diagnosed yearly. In North America alone, ten million people are now living with cancer and 600,000 people will die of it this year. To understand the scope of the tragedy, imagine that the evening newscast reported the no-survivors-crash of four fully loaded Boeing 747s every day, or the toll in human lives represented

FEARS..... AND REALITY	
Perceived threat	**Actual risk**
Terrorist attack	Infinitesimal (too small to be calculated)
Death in a shark attack	1 in 280,000,000
Death in an airplane crash	1 in 3,000,000
Death by lightning	1 in 350,000
Death in a motor vehicle accident	1 in 7,000
Food poisoning	1 in 7
Cardiovascular illness	1 in 4
Premature death related to obesity	1 in 4
Cancer	1 in 3
Death as a result of smoking (in smokers)	1 in 2

Source: Time magazine   **Figure 1**

in the fall of the Twin Towers of the World Trade Center in New York three times a week. That's without taking into account the costs associated with treatment for people with cancer, estimated to be 180 billion dollars annually – a price tag that will not stop growing in the foreseeable future. These figures illustrate the scale of the public health problem posed by cancer and highlight the need of identifying new ways of reducing the negative impact of this disease on society.

Beyond the statistics, cancer is first of all a human tragedy that strikes and kills people who are precious and dear to us, a disease that deprives young children of their mothers and fathers, that leaves an open wound in the lives of parents heartbroken by the death of their child. The loss of loved ones provokes an immense feeling of injustice and anger, the feeling of having lived through a trial brought on by a stroke of bad luck, an unhappy accident of fate that strikes at random and from which one cannot escape. Not only does cancer destroy human lives, it instills in us a profound doubt about our ability to conquer it.

We can fight cancer through diet

This feeling of helplessness in the face of cancer is reflected by polls taken to learn more about public opinion about the causes of this disease. In general, people see cancer as a disease triggered by uncontrollable factors: 89 percent of those recently polled believe that cancer occurs in those who are genetically predisposed toward it; furthermore, 80 percent consider that environmental factors (such as industrial pollution or pesticide residues present in non-organically grown food) are also important causes of cancer. A stunning majority (92 percent) associate smoking with cancer. However, less than half of the population considers that their eating habits might influence their risk of developing the disease. Overall, these impressions suggest that people are generally fatalistic about the possibility of preventing cancer, something that appears very unlikely or even impossible to half of them.

Every individual concerned with public health should be worried about the results of these polls and should consider the need to re-examine the communication strategies designed to inform people about the causes of cancer. Why? Because with the exception of smoking, people's perceptions are completely at odds with what the scientific community has succeeded in identifying as triggers for cancer.

As we look at the causes of cancer, you will discover that a minority of cancers are caused by factors that really cannot be controlled (**see Figure 2, below**). For example, hereditary factors are an important cause of cancer; they do not, however, play the fundamental role that people assign them. Current studies, especially those following sets of identical twins, indicate that a maximum of 15 percent of cancers are caused by malfunctioning genes and are therefore transmitted by heredity. The gap between the actual causes of cancer and popular belief is even greater when considering pollution-related causes, since, far from being a decisive factor in the development of cancer, exposure to air and water pollution, as well as exposure to pesticide residues, in fact represents barely 2 percent of all cases of cancer.

We can blame, and rightly so, the many harmful consequences of these environmental

RISK FACTORS FOR CANCER

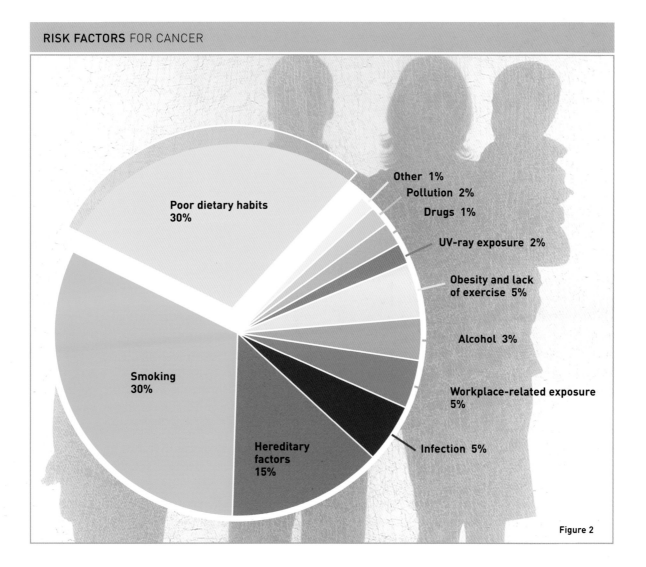

Poor dietary habits
30%

Other 1%
Pollution 2%
Drugs 1%

UV-ray exposure 2%

Obesity and lack
of exercise 5%

Alcohol 3%

Smoking
30%

Workplace-related exposure
5%

Infection 5%

Hereditary
factors
15%

Figure 2

factors, but atmospheric pollution has much more of an impact on ecosystem equilibrium than it does on the incidence of cancer. The same is true for pesticide residues associated with the fruits and vegetables we buy at the market. These pesticides are present in infinitesimally small quantities and no study has ever shown that they might cause cancer in such small doses. On the contrary, as we will see throughout this book, the consumption of fruits and vegetables has been associated over and over again with a decreased risk of developing cancer; so much so, in fact, that the benefits of including these foods in one's diet far outweigh the small risk linked to the presence of tiny quantities of pesticides.

In general, the risk factors that are difficult to control – those of hereditary, environmental or viral origin – are responsible for about 30 percent of all cancers (see Figure 2, p.15). Conversely, many factors directly related to lifestyle choices, such as smoking, lack of physical activity, obesity, and dietary habits, as well as the immoderate use of alcohol and drugs, are the direct cause of the onset of about 70 percent of all cancers!

It is important to call into question our false perceptions about cancer-causing agents, since this allows us to confront our defeatist attitude toward the disease and attack the problem from a new angle. If two-thirds of cancers are caused by factors outside of our genetic makeup and are related instead to our lifestyle habits, doesn't this imply that we can avoid two in three cancers simply by changing the way we live?

A MAP OF CANCER

One example of the profound influence of lifestyle choices on the development of cancer is spectacularly illustrated by studying the distribution of cancer cases on the planet (see Figure 3, opposite). Cancer doesn't seem to be evenly distributed throughout the world! According to the latest statistics published by the World Health Organization, the countries with the highest incidence of cancer are those in Eastern Europe (such as Hungary and the Czech Republic) with 300 to 400 cases per 100,000 inhabitants, closely followed by Western industrialized nations, such as the United States and Canada, with 260 cases per 100,000 inhabitants. Southeast Asian nations, such as India, China, and Thailand, have much lower rates – about 100 cases per 100,000 inhabitants.

Distribution of cancer types

Not only is the cancer burden unevenly distributed from one region of the globe to another, but the type of cancers affecting the population of different countries varies greatly. As a general rule, with the exception of lung cancer, which is the most frequently occurring and the most uniformly distributed cancer on the planet (due to smoking), the most common cancers occurring in Western industrialized nations are completely different from those affecting Asian countries. In the United States and Canada, in addition to lung cancer, the principal cancers are, in order of importance, colorectal cancer, breast cancer, and prostate cancer, while the frequency of these cancers in Asian countries is much lower than stomach, esophageal, and liver cancers.

The scale of these differences between East and West is striking; for example, in certain areas of the United States, over 100 women in 100,000 develop breast cancer; only 8 in 100,000 Thai women are so afflicted. The situation is similar for colon cancer: while people in some areas of North America have a colon cancer incidence of

50 per 100,000 inhabitants, only 8 in 100,000 Indians contract the disease. With prostate cancer, the other major killer in Western societies, the difference is even more telling: this cancer afflicts ten times fewer Japanese and up to one hundred times fewer Thai men than Westerners.

The study of migrant populations has allowed us to confirm that these extreme variations are not due to any random genetic predisposition; rather, that they are intimately linked to lifestyle differences. **Table 1 on p.18** shows a striking example of the variations due to emigration. In the study illustrated here, the levels of different cancers affecting Japanese and Japanese immigrants to Hawaii were compared with those affecting the ethnic Hawaiian population. For example, while prostate cancer was at the time little-known in Japan, the incidence of this cancer increased by a factor of 10 in Japanese immigrants to Hawaii, to the point of becoming comparable to the native Hawaiian levels. Conversely, the high levels of stomach cancer characteristic of native Japanese and caused by infection with *Helicobacter pylori* bacteria, diminished considerably and also began to approach native-born Hawaiian levels. Similar phenomena are observed in Japanese women, whose low rates of breast and uterine cancer increase markedly when they change their lifestyle upon leaving Japan for the West.

These statistics do not constitute an isolated case, far from it: very similar results have been obtained by studying different populations all over the globe. We will note one further

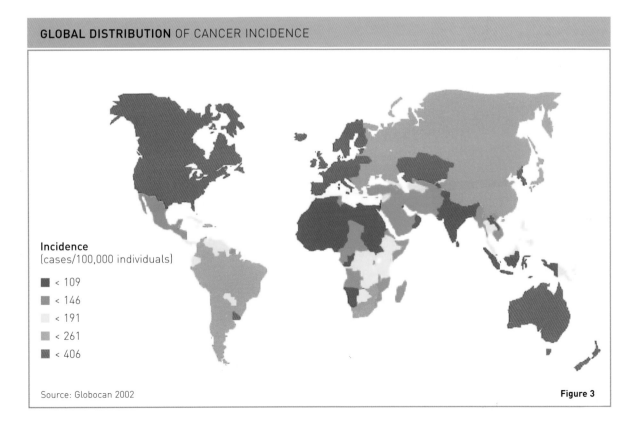

GLOBAL DISTRIBUTION OF CANCER INCIDENCE

Incidence
(cases/100,000 individuals)

■ < 109
■ < 146
■ < 191
■ < 261
■ < 406

Source: Globocan 2002

Figure 3

example, which compares the rates of certain types of cancers in African–Americans with those in Nigerians (**see Table 2, opposite**). Yet again, the Nigerians in the study showed cancer levels that were radically different from those of the African–Americans. Prostate cancer rates are much higher in the United States, while the opposite was observed for the rate of liver cancer, which is much greater in Africa due to the prevalence there of the principal cause of primary cancer in this organ, the hepatitis virus. In any case, the cancer rate in the African–American population is almost identical to that in Caucasian Americans, and completely different from that in their Black African counterparts. These studies are extremely interesting: in addition to offering irrefutable proof that most cancers are not in fact due to hereditary factors, they point to the preponderant role played by lifestyle in the development of this disease.

But what lifestyle modification could have such a devastating influence on the health of these immigrant populations, to the point of inducing such a rapid increase in cancer rates? All the studies carried out to this day point to a specific culprit: the abandoning of traditional dietary practices coupled with a rapid adaptation to the host country's culinary habits. In the two cases described here, the changes are dramatic:

COMPARISON OF THE INCIDENCE OF CANCER AS A FUNCTION OF PRIMARY LOCATION IN NATIVE-BORN JAPANESE LIVING IN JAPAN AND IMMIGRANT CAUCASIANS AND JAPANESE LIVING IN HAWAII

ANNUAL INCIDENCE/MILLION INDIVIDUALS

Primary cancer location	Japan	Hawaiian Japanese	Hawaiian Caucasians
Esophagus	131	46	75
Stomach	1,311	397	217
Colon	83	371	368
Rectum	93	297	204
Lung	268	379	962
Prostate	14	154	343
Breast	315	1,221	1,869
Cervix	364	149	243
Uterus	26	407	714
Ovary	53	160	274

Source: Doll, R., and Peto, R. (1981) J. Natl. Cancer Inst. 66, 1196-1305.   **Table 1**

Japanese immigrants to the West left behind an exemplary diet, one rich in complex carbohydrates and vegetables and low in fat, for a diet containing large amounts of proteins and animal fat.

In fact, even without the question of emigration, Japanese dietary habits in the last fifty years have undergone huge changes that also illustrate the role of diet in the onset of cancer. For example, a mere forty years ago the consumption of meat was relatively low in Japan; it has increased by a factor of seven in recent years, and the rate of colon cancer is now five times what it was, matching that of the West. It is therefore extremely interesting,

although a little alarming, to realize the degree to which the adoption of Western habits and practices has caused an increase in the rate of certain cancers.

THE IMPACT OF DIET ON CANCER

We now estimate that 30 percent of all cancers are directly related to the type of diet favored by different individuals. This huge percentage may seem surprising, since the foods we consume on a daily basis might not appear to be a risk factor as important as, say, smoking. Nonetheless, as we have seen from the previous data, changes in diet have a real impact on the risk of developing a very large number of cancers. In fact, the

COMPARISON OF THE INCIDENCE OF CANCER AS A FUNCTION OF PRIMARY LOCATION IN THE INHABITANTS OF IBADAN (NIGERIA), AFRICAN–AMERICANS, AND CAUCASIAN AMERICANS

ANNUAL INCIDENCE/MILLION INDIVIDUALS

Primary cancer location	Ibadan	African–Americans	Caucasian Americans
Colon	34	351	315
Rectum	34	204	225
Liver	272	77	36
Pancreas	55	225	124
Larynx	37	193	141
Prostate	134	651	275
Lung	27	1,532	981
Breast	337	1,187	1,650
Uterus	42	407	714
Lymphosarcoma	133	7	4

Source: Doll, R., and Peto, R. (1981) J. Natl. Cancer Inst. 66, 1196-1305.   **Table 2**

proportion of deaths due to cancer that is directly linked to diet may reach 90 percent in the case of cancers affecting the gastrointestinal system (the esophagus, stomach, and colon)!

What is it in the diet, exactly, that exerts such an important influence on the chance of developing cancer? Several factors are responsible, but some more than most: recent epidemiological studies have succeeded in establishing a close relationship between the lack of fruits and vegetables in the diet and an increase in the rate of certain cancers. The results obtained in over 200 of these studies are spectacular (see Table 3, below): 80 percent show that a significant intake of fruits and vegetables leads to a marked decrease in the risk

of developing cancer; this effect was especially notable in cancers of the digestive system. In general, individuals consuming the fewest fruits and vegetables have around twice the chance of developing certain cancers than people who consume greater quantities of these foods.

Since diet in Western societies and particularly in North America is generally characterized by the relative absence of fruits and vegetables, the results of these studies suggest that these dietary shortcomings could play a role in the higher cancer rates now afflicting the West. This is the reason that North American and European public health documents, such as the FDA's Food Guide Pyramid, recommend eating at least five servings of fruits and vegetables every day

EPIDEMIOLOGICAL STUDIES ON THE RELATIONSHIP BETWEEN FRUITS AND VEGETABLES AND THE DEVELOPMENT OF CANCER

Food studied	Observation of a decrease in risk	Total number of studies	Percentage (%) of studies suggesting a decrease in risk
Vegetables in general	59	74	80
Fruits in general	36	56	64
Raw vegetables	40	46	87
Cruciferous vegetables (broccoli, cabbage...)	38	55	69
Allium family vegetables (garlic, onions, leeks...)	27	35	77
Green vegetables	68	88	77
Carrots	59	73	81
Tomatoes	36	51	71
Citrus fruit	27	41	66

Source: World Cancer Research Fund/American Institute for Cancer Research, 1997   **Table 3**

as part of a varied and balanced diet that is intended to maintain good health.

The East–West divide

To understand how diet might contribute to the differences observed in the respective rates of cancers in the East and the West, we must first note that these two broadly defined cultures have perceptions of the place of food in daily life that are diametrically opposed to one another. In the West, where eating is perceived above all as an act designed to supply the body with the energy needed for survival, we generally describe food as a source of calories and vitamins. In Asia, however, diet has always been associated with the preservation of health; the consumption of foods essential in satisfying energy needs does not occur to the detriment of physical and mental wellbeing.

Since energy supply is the main objective pursued by Western diet, we should not be surprised that the latter is based for the most part on the consumption of proteins and animal fats, such as red meat and dairy products, while foods with fewer calories, such as fruits and vegetables, occupy a place of less importance. In the East, people consume fruits and vegetables in abundance; their main sources of protein are legumes, particularly soybeans, as well as fish; they eat relatively little red meat and other foods containing saturated animal fats.

In addition to this imbalance tipped in favor of saturated fats, many characteristics of the Western diet are puzzling when one considers their impact on health. We may well acknowledge the considerable and undeniable positive effects of industrialization and technological advances on lifestyle, but the repercussions of industrialization on the nature and quality of foods available to consumers are completely catastrophic. Western consumers are confronted on a daily basis with an avalanche of processed foods prepared on an industrial scale using poor-quality ingredients.

How industrialization has affected our food

The flour used in preparing breads and pasta is often bleached, refined, and far too finely ground: eating these products leads to the quick release of sugar to the bloodstream. Vegetable oils can be treated with hydrogen, which changes their chemical makeup by hardening them, thereby creating potentially toxic fats, such as trans-fats. Many products such as cured and smoked foods contain preservatives that may be converted into carcinogenic substances in the body. The pervasive witch hunt that has recently targeted all types of fats has led to the production of foods so tasteless and lacking in interest that huge amounts of sugar must be added to give them some kind of flavor.

Unfortunately, people prepare their own meals less and less often and turn to these products as quick substitutes, thus limiting the possibility of controlling the content of their diet. The consequence of the industrialization of food is that the contemporary Western diet has almost nothing in common with what made up the essence of human diet scarcely ten generations ago. The modern diet contains at least twice as much fat, a much higher percentage of saturated fat relative to unsaturated fat, barely a third of the fiber, an avalanche of sugar in place of complex carbohydrates and, paradoxically, reduced amounts of essential nutrients when compared to a traditional diet.

Another perverse effect of the industrialization of food is large-scale production, using methods that justify higher production costs and that make food abundantly available and affordable for the great majority of people. However, this very abundance incites many people to eat too much and badly, loading their bodies with fats and sugar. One of the most serious consequences of the overconsumption of fats and sugar is that the caloric surplus that results leads directly to obesity. During the period when the "anti-fat" creed was most in vogue, between 1980 and 2000, the percentage of obese Americans more than doubled, rising from 12 to 28 percent of the population; no fewer than 65 percent of Americans are now overweight. These statistics are dramatic, since obesity is accompanied by a contingent of cardiovascular diseases, type 2 diabetes, retinopathies (diseases of the retina), respiratory ailments, and other health problems, all associated with excess body weight.

Obesity and cancer

Even though the media have begun to familiarize their audience with the problems linked to obesity, not enough people are aware that obesity constitutes in and of itself the most important dietary risk factor in developing cancer. A recent American study carried out on 900,000 overweight people showed a marked increase in the risk of developing certain types of cancers, such as endometrial cancer, breast cancer, and colon cancer, in these subjects. Obesity is considered today to be responsible for 35 percent of deaths linked to colon cancer in men and, alarmingly, almost 60 percent of deaths caused by endometrial cancer in women. In other words, a body mass index or BMI (your weight in kilograms divided by the square of your height in meters) of over 25 may be responsible for 10 percent of all deaths linked to cancer in American non-smokers.

As we have observed, Japanese immigrants to the West have seen their risk of contracting certain types of cancers, such as those of the breast and the prostate, increase by a factor of ten. We also observe that European and Asian nations that have changed their dietary traditions to accommodate eating habits imported from North America have been hit by a stunning increase in levels of obesity and colon and prostate cancer, as well as cardiovascular disease, which were all previously relatively rare in these areas.

Despite these alarming statistics, junk food and fast food advertising remains sadly ubiquitous and targets, tragically, an ever younger public of children and adolescents. We tend to accept this marketing onslaught with remarkable passivity: meals made up of huge hamburgers and gallons of carbonated soft drinks, potato chips loaded with trans-fats and acrylamide fats, and other "snack" foods that constantly appear on our television screens during prime time. Accepting this kind of advertising is tantamount to resigning ourselves to spending considerable sums on health care for future generations. We absolutely must stop considering food as nothing but fuel and eating as an act designed solely to satisfy cravings that has no impact at all on our health.

Alternatives to the Western diet

There is thus no doubt that radically modifying our diet must be the inescapable goal of any preventive strategy designed to reduce the number of cancers affecting Western societies. Fortunately, more and more people wishing to change their dietary habits can now count on an ever-increasing number of products of excellent quality, made with healthy ingredients, that can really contribute to better overall health. Many major supermarkets now include a section where these foods are prominently featured, not to mention the numerous markets where we can familiarize ourselves with typical ingredients and products from culinary traditions the world over, most of which were completely unknown to us only thirty years ago. In fact, if globalization has had unfortunate repercussions for people who switched to a Western way of life, Westerners can benefit from the culinary traditions of other cultures. For those who wish to eat healthily and protect themselves against diseases as deadly as cancer, an alternative to Western junk food exists.

How this book can help

The object of this book is not to promote a specific diet or diets; we believe that there are excellent books available on the subject (**see Bibliography, p.185**). These books contain all the relevant information on the ways of obtaining a balanced intake of proteins, fats, and carbohydrates, as well as vitamins and minerals. We wish to bring something else to the table, as it were: the perspective of scientists interested in the role played by diet in the development of cancer and in publicizing foods that may indeed help reduce the risk of developing this disease.

The recommendations in this book are based on the well-established role of fruits and vegetables as the essential components in any diet designed to fight cancer, but they also take into account new scientific data that suggest that the very nature of fruits and vegetables plays as significant a role as the amounts consumed, since certain foods constitute an exceptional source of anticancer molecules. In the course of the last five years, our research laboratory has become

interested in the identification of anticancer molecules present in these foods, as well as in understanding the mechanisms by which these molecules prevent the development of cancer. This work has allowed us to identify several anticancer molecules of dietary origin, but the results obtained have been published only in specialized journals; the real benefits that these foods may have in cancer prevention and in public health remain little known overall.

Our project was conceived in this spirit. We wanted to write a book in layman's terms that described the scientific data demonstrating the crucial role of diet in the development of cancer, so that the greatest possible number of people could benefit from the most recent discoveries. We hope to communicate to you our belief that a diet based on the regular intake of the right foods is indispensable to fighting cancer.

In summary

● **Individual lifestyle** choices play a major role in the risk of developing cancer.

● **Approximately one-third** of all cancers are directly related to diet.

● **Enjoying a diverse,** balanced diet, rich in fruits and vegetables, coupled with controlled calorie intake to avoid weight gain, is a simple and effective way of significantly reducing the risk of developing cancer.

"Know your enemy and know yourself; had you then a hundred wars to fight, you would be a hundred times victorious."

Sun Tzu, *The Art of War*

What is Cancer?

The development of cancer takes place over a long period of time and involves many complex processes. However, the basic mechanism of cancer is not difficult to understand. Knowing how cancer arises can help you understand how some foods may help prevent this terrible disease.

THE NATURE OF THE ENEMY

In spite of decades of dedicated and determined research, financed to the tune of billions of dollars, a large number of cancers remain impossible to treat; even when specific treatment is available for some types of cancers, the long-term patient survival rate is still too often lower than we might expect or are willing to accept. On many occasions, new drugs that inspired great enthusiasm have turned out to be less effective than predicted, and in some cases, not effective at all. What makes cancer so difficult to treat? This is a crucial question that must be addressed before we can touch on the new methods we hope to use in fighting this disease.

Of course, knowing one's enemy is very important, but please be reassured that it is not our intention to describe in an overly detailed manner all the molecular events that lead to tumor formation. We believe that this kind of description would only serve to emphasize the complexity of cancer, while failing to add anything new or useful to understanding the means at our disposal to reduce cancer rates. However, it is often possible to know the broad outlines of character and motivation, the strengths and weaknesses of an individual without necessarily knowing all the details of his or her life. This chapter has just such a goal in mind: to allow you to learn about the cancer cell by looking at only the broad outline of its "personality" and the motivation that drives it to invade surrounding tissues and grow to the point of threatening life itself, to discover what allows it to take hold, and, more importantly, to identify its weaknesses so as to better defend against it. This exercise might seem difficult to the reader unfamiliar with biology or science in general, but it is a very worthwhile one. Only when we understand what cancer is can we learn how dangerous and formidable an enemy it can be, an enemy that must be considered with a certain respect. It takes an understanding of what cancer is to learn how to exploit its weaknesses and keep it at a distance.

THE ROOT OF ALL EVIL: THE CELL

The cell is the base unit of all life on Earth, from the humblest bacterium to more complex organisms such as human beings, who are made up of over 60,000 billion cells. This tiny structure, which measures from 10 to 100 μm (a micron is one one–thousandth of a millimeter), is one of Nature's most incredible masterpieces, a puzzle of stupefying complexity that continues to fascinate the scientists seeking to unlock its mysteries. Although the cell has not yet given up all its secrets, we now understand that a disturbance in its functioning may lead to the development of cancer. Thus, from a scientific point of view, cancer is first and foremost a disease of the cell.

To better understand the cell, we can compare it to a city where all the functions essential for the wellbeing of the community have been assigned to its different parts, so that all workers can benefit from optimal conditions in order to perform their tasks (**see Figure 4, below**).

The nucleus

Four principal constituents of the cell may be said to play a significant role when it comes to cancer. The first of these is the nucleus, which serves as the cell library, the area where the codebooks are stored: these are called genes, and they regulate the administration of the city. Cells contain about 25,000 laws, or codes, dispersed in the heart of a voluminous text, DNA, which is written in a strange alphabet composed of only four letters: A, T, C, and G. It is important to read these laws; they tell the cell how to behave by letting it make the proteins essential to its good working order and to its response to any change in its environment. For example, an alert that signals that the cell is about to need sugar is followed immediately by the reading, or enacting, of a law that authorizes the creation of new proteins specialized in sugar transportation,

---

DNA AND PROTEINS, MAESTROS OF CELL FUNCTION

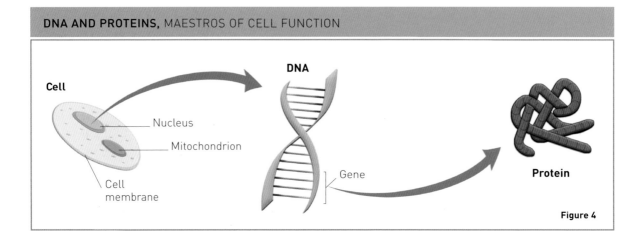

Cell
— Nucleus
— Mitochondrion
Cell membrane

DNA

Gene

Protein

Figure 4

which leads to the resolution of the crisis: re-establishment of sufficient sugar reserves to allow the cell to survive. When mistakes occur in the reading of the codes, the proteins that are formed are incapable of adequately fulfilling their function and may contribute instead to the formation of cancers.

Proteins

Proteins are the "workforce" of the city; they get the job done. These molecules take care of most of the necessary functions that maintain cell viability: the transport of nutrients through the bloodstream, the communication of messages sent from outside to inform the cell of changes in that outer realm, the process of nutrient conversion that produces energy, and so forth. Many proteins are enzymes, or the "artists" of the cell, since they possess the ability to transform unusable substances into compounds essential to the life of the cell. Some enzymes also allow the cell to adapt rapidly to any changes in the environment by subtly modifying the function of other proteins. It is thus essential for the cell always to make sure that the reading of the laws that govern the production of these enzymes is faithful to the original text; a bad reading might lead to the creation of proteins that are incapable of adequately performing their work and that act in a way that is incompatible with the equilibrium of the cell. Cancer is always caused by mistakes in protein production, and especially enzyme production.

The mitochondrion

The mitochondrion is the city's power plant, its energy center; it is the place where the energy contained in the structure of molecules derived from food (carbohydrates, proteins, lipids) is converted into cellular energy (ATP). Oxygen is used as fuel for this process, which results in the formation of toxic waste in the form of free radicals. This waste can trigger the formation of a tumor by introducing changes in the genes, leading to mistakes in protein production.

The cell membrane

The structure that surrounds the cell is made of lipids and certain proteins, and acts as a wall designed to contain all cell activities in one place. The cell membrane plays an extremely important role, since it acts as a barrier between the interior of the cell and what lies outside. It is a kind of filter that sorts out the substances that can enter the cell and those that can leave. The membrane contains several proteins called receptors that detect the chemical signals present in the bloodstream and transmit the messages coded by these signals to the cell, so that it can react to changes in environment. This function is a crucial one for the cell; we can understand why a misreading of the genes controlling the production of these proteins can have dramatic consequences. When a cell no longer understands what is going on outside its borders, it loses its bearings and starts to act autonomously, without paying attention to cells in its immediate vicinity. This is dangerous behavior; behavior that can lead to cancer.

THE CONSTRAINTS ON CELLS WHEN THEY WORK TOGETHER

So, what pushes a cell over the edge, causing it to become cancerous? Most people know that cancer is caused by excessive, uncontrolled cell growth, but as a general rule, the factors that promote the development of this behavior remain mysterious. As in any traditional psychological analysis, the answers are to be found in the cell's infancy.

The human cell as it now exists is the result of the evolution of a primitive cell that appeared on Earth about three and half billion years ago, looking more like a bacterium than the human cell that we know today. Over this long period, the ancestral cell was subjected to huge changes in its environment (UV rays, changes in oxygen levels, and so forth) that forced it to constantly seek out, by trial and error, the "right" modification, the one that would grant it the best chance of survival. The cell's great ability to adapt is due to its capacity for modifying its genes to allow for the production of new proteins that are more effective in facing new problems. We must understand that genes, those famous codebooks we have been discussing, are not immutable; as soon as a cell senses that it needs to modify the codebook to get around a tight spot, it will rewrite the code: this is known as a mutation. This ability that cells have to mutate their genes is thus an essential characteristic of life, without which we would simply not exist.

The origins of multicellular organisms

About 600 million years ago, cells made a "decision" that had the most far-reaching consequences in evolutionary history on Earth: they began to cohabit, thus forming the first multicellular organisms. This was a radical event in the very "mentality" of the cell, since cohabitation implies that the survival of the organism takes precedence over that of individual cells. The constant search for improving in order to better adapt to changes in cell environment could thus no longer be done at the expense of the organism's other cells. In other words, formerly individualistic cells gradually became altruistic, in a way renouncing their fundamental freedom to transform their

genes at will. This evolutionary change remained, since it brought with it many advantages, the most important of which was that different cells could now participate in a division of labor: cells could divide tasks among themselves in order to better interact with the environment. For example, in a primitive organism certain cells developed an expertise in tasks related to the identification of nutrients present in their immediate environment, while others specialized in digesting food so as to obtain energy for the organism. To reach this stage of specialization, cells had to change their laws (the codebooks) so that they could form new kinds of proteins that improved their performance and allowed them to accomplish their tasks that much more efficiently; they had to learn to get along. This ability to adapt is the basis for evolution; but in the case of multicellular organisms, the adaptation that occurs must benefit the entire organism and not just an individual cell.

In human beings, cell specialization has attained a peak of complexity. In fact, it is difficult to imagine that a skin (epithelial) cell, for example, might in some way be related to a kidney cell, or that muscle cells have a common origin with the neurons that let us think. Nevertheless, all cells in the human body do possess the same genetic baggage, the same codes in their nuclei. If an epithelial cell differs from a kidney cell, it's not because these two types of cells don't have the same genes, but rather because they don't use the same genes to accomplish their respective functions. In other words, each human cell uses only those genes

▶ **Healthy cells** in human skin "know" the role they must play and are able to act together. If they "forget" their role and act independently, cancer can arise.

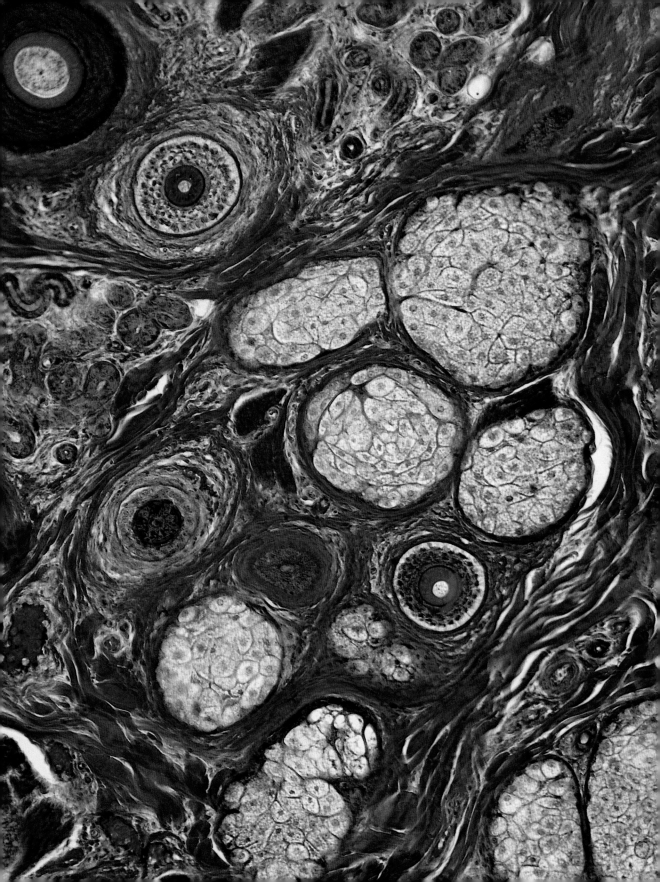

that are compatible with its function. This phenomenon is called cellular differentiation. Maintaining cellular differentiation is critical to the optimal functioning of the organism; if our neurons suddenly decided to behave as if they were epithelial cells and stopped transmitting nerve impulses, the entire organism would suffer. The same is true for any one of our organs – each type of cell must carry out the task that it has been assigned for the wellbeing of all of the organism's cells. When we stop to reflect that the human body contains 60,000 billion (60 trillion) cells that all have to listen to one another, we can only be amazed at the order inherent in such a complex structure.

THE SUICIDAL TENDENCIES OF CELLS

The body has worked out an extremely detailed and rigorous program to retire damaged or non-functioning cells: ritual suicide! Apoptosis allows the organism to destroy a cell in a "clean" manner without causing damage to surrounding cells or bringing about inflammatory reactions in tissue. This is an essential phenomenon that is part of many physiological processes: embryonic development, the elimination of incompetent immune system cells, and the destruction of cells that present significant damage to their DNA. This final point is a crucial one when considering cancer.

WHEN CELLS REBEL

If the adequate functioning of an organism as complex as the human being requires the complete repression of the ancestral survival instincts of cells, as well as the combining of all their resources, we can easily imagine that maintaining these functions is a fragile phenomenon, one constantly subjected to attempts at "rebellion" by cells who wish to

---

RULES FOR CELLS

1 Reproduction is not permitted, except in order to replace a dead or damaged cell.

2 Staying alive is not permitted if damage is detected in the structure of the cell, particularly at the DNA level. If the damage is too great, suicide is mandatory!

---

recover some freedom of action. This is exactly what happens throughout our lives: when a cell is subjected to outside aggression, caused by a carcinogenic substance, a virus, or by an excess of free radicals, its first reflex is to interpret the aggression as an ordeal that it must cope with as best it can: by mutating its genes so as to get around the obstacle.

Unfortunately for us, these aggressions are common over the course of our lives; some cells damaged in these attacks become fed up and rebel, forgetting their essential role as part of the organism as a whole. It is in the organism's interest to prevent the damaged cell from gaining too much autonomy; the "good will" of cells is strictly controlled by a set of rules that ensure that the cell's code of social behavior is always obeyed. Fortunately, this allows for the rapid destruction of any rebel cells, thereby ensuring that the body is able to maintain its vital functions.

However, these rules are not perfectly enforced, and some cells manage to complete the gene mutations that will let them get around the rules, and form a tumor. In other words, a cancer occurs when a cell stops playing the role that was assigned to it and refuses to cooperate with other cells in order to guarantee the smooth functioning of the organism as a whole. That cell becomes an outlaw isolated from other cells that refuses to respond to the orders transmitted by the society of which it is a member. It has only one purpose: to ensure its own survival and that of its offspring. All bets are now off: the rebel cell has reclaimed its ancestral survival instincts.

THE ONSET OF CANCER

It is important to understand that this transformation of the cell does not necessarily mean that a cancer will immediately develop in the organism. Later on in this book, we shall see that this delinquent cell behavior happens regularly over an individual's lifespan, without necessarily leading to cancer. The growth of cancer should rather be seen as a gradual phenomenon, able to evolve quietly and anonymously over many years, or even decades, before symptoms appear. This "slowness" to develop is extremely important for us, because,

as this book will make clear, it gives us a golden opportunity to intervene at any one of the many stages of tumor development and to block the evolution of the rebel cell into a mature cancer cell. Although each cancer has its own triggering events, all cancers follow the same broad development process, with three major stages: initiation, promotion, and progression (see Figure 5, below).

Stage one: Initiation

As its name indicates, initiation is the first stage of carcinogenesis (cancer growth), where the exposure of cells to a carcinogenic substance triggers irreversible damage to cell DNA and leads to the appearance of a mutation. Many things, such as ultraviolet rays, certain viruses, cigarette smoke, or carcinogenic substances in the food we eat can all cause this damage and initiate the cancer.

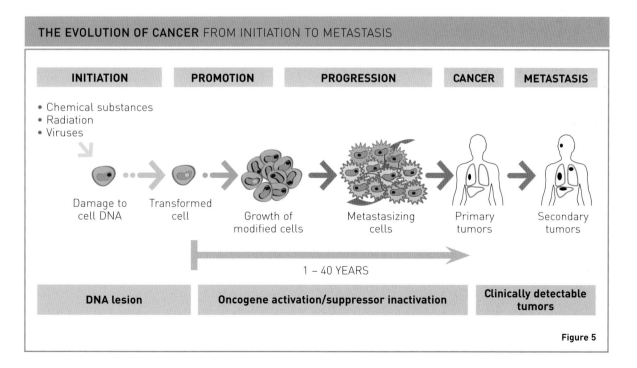

THE EVOLUTION OF CANCER FROM INITIATION TO METASTASIS

| INITIATION | PROMOTION | PROGRESSION | CANCER | METASTASIS |

- Chemical substances
- Radiation
- Viruses

Damage to cell DNA → Transformed cell → Growth of modified cells → Metastasizing cells → Primary tumors → Secondary tumors

1 – 40 YEARS

| DNA lesion | Oncogene activation/suppressor inactivation | Clinically detectable tumors |

Figure 5

THE SIX SIGNATURE TRACES OF CANCER

1 Anarchic growth: cancer cells reproduce themselves in the absence of chemical signals.

2 The refusal to obey the order to stop growth that is given by nearby cells that perceive the danger to surrounding tissue.

3 Resistance to cellular suicide by apoptosis, which allows the cells to bypass the control of the cell's protection mechanisms.

4 The ability to form new blood vessels by angiogenesis, allowing the oxygen and nutrients necessary for growth to reach the cell.

5 Immortality: the acquisition of all of these characteristics causes the cancerous cells to become immortal, capable of infinite reproduction.

6 The ability to invade and colonize the organism's tissues, first locally, and then more widely, through the spread of metastasized cells.

However, at this stage (with a few exceptions), the "initiated" cells are not sufficiently activated for us to call them cancerous; they can only potentially form tumors, if the exposure to the toxic agent continues regularly or if a factor in promotion allows the initiated cell to pursue its new path, trying to find new mutations that might help it develop on its own. As we shall see, certain molecules present in foods have the property of keeping these potential tumors in a dormant state and may thus prevent cancer from developing.

Stage two: Promotion

During this stage, the initiated cell ignores the two rules for cells given on p.30 and attains the critical threshold of the transformed cell. A good deal of ongoing cancer research now focuses on the identification of factors that allow cells to bypass the cell's usual rules.

Generally, in order to get past rule one, cancer cells produce large amounts of proteins that allow cells to grow autonomously, without outside help. In parallel fashion, a cell on the path to becoming cancerous must rid itself of the proteins responsible for the application of rule two, without which all of its efforts would be immediately countered by the mechanism of cellular suicide known as apoptosis. In both cases, the mutations that trigger a modification in protein function lead to the uncontrolled growth of the modified cells. However, this is a difficult stage, which takes place over a long period of time, sometimes up to forty years, since the cell must make multiple attempts at mutation in the hope of acquiring the characteristics necessary for its growth.

The factors that promote cell disobedience with respect to the two rules of cell behavior are still poorly understood, but it is possible that hormones, those important growth factors, as well as free radical levels, all play a role at this crucial stage. Nevertheless, we can surmise that the promotion stage offers the largest window of opportunity that we have to intervene if we wish to prevent the onset of cancer, since many of the factors involved can be mostly controlled by the lifestyle of individuals.

As we shall see in detail in subsequent chapters, there is no doubt that many factors of dietary origin can have a positive impact on the situation by keeping the future tumor at this premature stage. This prevention is very important, because the transformed cells that succeed in getting by the first two stages become extremely dangerous, and are set to become even more dangerous in the course of the next stage, which is known as progression.

Stage three: Progression

It is in the course of the third stage that the transformed cell gains its independence, as well as characteristics that are more and more malignant and that help it begin to invade the tissue in which it is localized. Stage three cells become metastasizing cells. All tumors that have succeeded in reaching the progression stage possess six common characteristics that may be considered as a kind of "signature" of the mature cancer (**see box, opposite**).

THE CHANCE TO STOP CANCER DEVELOPING

We have seen that the appearance of a tumor is not an instantaneous phenomenon. Rather, it is the result of a long process that takes place over several years, when the cell, "awakened" by contact with a carcinogenic substance, transforms itself to overcome the many obstacles that threatened it at every stage of its development. The most important point of this long process is that, for many years, or even decades, the cancerous cells remain very vulnerable; only a few of them will succeed in reaching the malignant stage. This vulnerability makes it possible for us to intervene and interfere at several stages of the process of tumor development, thus preventing the onset of the disease. We shall come back to this point throughout this book, because it is such a crucial aspect of any strategy of reducing cancer mortality: the tumor must be attacked while it is vulnerable if we really want the death rate from cancer in our society to decrease. By rediscovering, so to speak, the primitive, ancestral instincts that assured its

autonomous, independent survival, the tumor cell becomes very formidable. This is what makes cancer so difficult to fight: trying to destroy these primitive cells is like trying to snuff out the very adaptation skills and strengths that allowed us originally to evolve into what we are now. It means trying to destroy the forces that lie at the very heart of life.

In summary

- Cancer is a disease caused by a disturbance in cellular function. Over the course of the malfunction, the cell progressively acquires certain defining characteristics that allow it to grow and invade surrounding tissue.

- The acquisition of these cancerous properties generally takes place over a long period of time, a latency period that gives us a golden opportunity to intervene in order to prevent the tumor from reaching the stage of maturity.

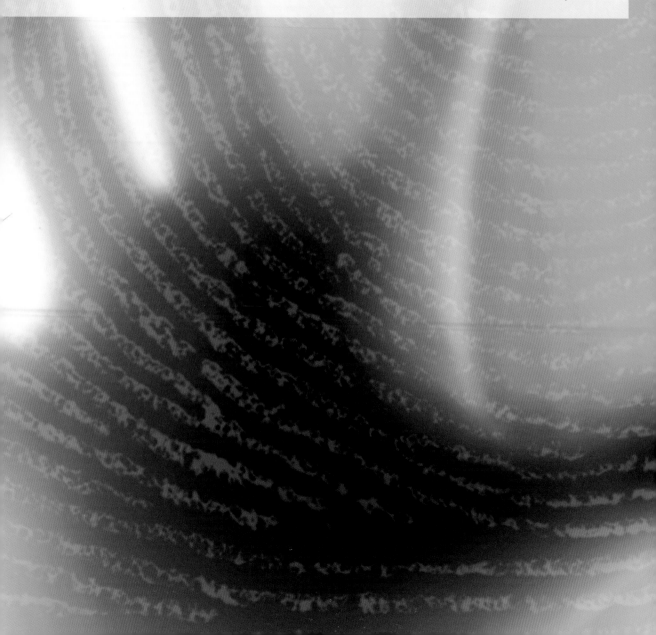

"Reduce the hostile chiefs by inflicting damage on them, and make trouble for them, and keep them constantly engaged..."

Sun Tzu, *The Art of War*

Preventing Cancer Growth

The mainstays of treating established cancer are surgery, radiotherapy, and chemotherapy, which all act to destroy malignant tumors. New approaches to cancer involve preventing cancer growth by attacking the tumor's blood supply, rather than the tumor itself, depriving it of food and keeping it at bay.

THE TREATMENT OF CANCER: CURRENT APPROACHES

If, as we have just seen, cancer cells have already evolved in order to confront many obstacles and have, in the process, become extremely resistant, we should not be surprised that cancer remains a disease that is very difficult to treat, especially when the diagnosis of the tumor occurs at a late stage after the cancer is well established. Considerable progress in the treatment of many cancers has been made over the last few years, mostly thanks to the development of new drugs and procedures that help detect tumors at early stages. However, very large variations exist in treatment success rates according to type of cancer. Although the cure rate (measured by the absence of tumor recurrence after five years) for breast cancer or prostate cancer can reach 70 percent, cancers of the lung, pancreas, and esophagus give few chances to those who have them, with survival rates not exceeding 20 percent. Globally, it is estimated that on average, only 60 percent of all cancer patients are still alive after five years.

Unlike other diseases, there is no universal procedure used to treat cancer. The type of cancer, its size, and its location in the body, as well as the nature of its cells at a particular point in time (what is commonly known as the "stage") and the overall health status of the patient, all represent important parameters in the choice of the best and most appropriate treatment strategy. There are now three broad categories of treatment: removal of the tumor by surgery, radiotherapy, and chemotherapy. A common current treatment procedure follows the surgical excision of the tumor with radiotherapy or chemotherapy to destroy residual cancer cells.

Surgery

Traditionally, surgery was the first weapon used against cancer; even today, it is often the front-line treatment, especially if the tumor is well localized and has been diagnosed at an early stage. The goal of surgery is to remove the entire tumor, or, in some cases, the entire affected organ. The major limit of surgery is that it cannot eliminate all cancerous cells in the body, especially the microfoci containing small undetectable tumors.

Radiotherapy

The goal of radiotherapy is to destroy cancerous cells by subjecting them to X-rays or high-energy gamma rays. Radiotherapy is a local treatment, applied on a precise, directed area so as to preserve as much healthy tissue as possible, since radiation will also kill normal cells. This method of treating cancer is very commonly used; about half of all North American cancer patients will be treated using radiotherapy, usually in conjunction with surgery and chemotherapy.

Chemotherapy

Chemotherapy is the treatment that inspires the greatest fear in cancer patients; it is generally perceived in a negative manner, mostly because of the many side effects patients may experience. However, despite its many undesirable effects, chemotherapy is the oncologist's weapon of choice, since intravenous administration allows medication to reach cancerous cells that are dispersed throughout the organism, which is impossible in surgery or with radiotherapy.

All drugs used in chemotherapy are extremely powerful cellular poisons that kill cells by preventing them from reproducing. Because cancer cells reproduce more often than normal cells, chemotherapy allows for the eradication of cancer cells with minimum impact on healthy ones. However, certain healthy cells, such as those that make up the intestinal lining or those in bone marrow, must also divide regularly to adequately fulfill their function; these cells are also prime targets for chemotherapy drugs, a phenomenon that contributes significantly to their toxic effects.

THE LIMITS OF CURRENT THERAPIES

In spite of the important progress made in treating the disease in the last few years, we must admit that cancer remains a public health problem of the first degree and that the means used to treat it are still all too often inadequate. The two major limits to current cancer therapies are the following:

Side effects

One of the great failings of chemotherapy medications is their toxicity to many normal, healthy cells; this toxicity is responsible for their many side effects. Among them, we can cite the drop in immune cell levels and blood platelets, anemia, digestive problems (nausea, inflammation of the gastric mucosa), and hair loss (alopecia), without mentioning the various heart, kidney, or other complications. As a consequence, the duration of chemotherapy treatment is often limited by the severity of the side effects and does not always allow for the complete elimination of the cancer cells. Also, certain chemotherapy drugs used in the treatment of many tumors cause mutations in the patient's DNA; these drugs are in and of themselves carcinogenic and may increase the risk of cancer in the long term.

Resistance

If the use of chemotherapy drugs constitutes an improvement in the treatment of certain types of cancer, even taking side effects into account, it is nonetheless true that many cancers cannot be cured in this way. This may seem surprising when one considers what powerful cell poisons these agents are, but the fact remains: cancer treatment faces its greatest obstacle in the form of the body's own resistance to cancer treatment.

Even though, as a general rule, all cancers are strongly diminished in size and number through the effects of chemotherapy (we say that these tumors "respond" to treatment), all too often a tumor will recur over time. These recurrences are generally bad news, since the new tumors have developed a resistance not only to the drug used in the initial treatment, but in some cases to other drugs as well. As we saw in the preceding chapter, cancer cells that have reached the tumor stage are extremely versatile and are capable of adapting themselves to a variety of hostile conditions.

During chemotherapy, a mechanism often used by tumor cells to adapt to the poison is to create proteins that "pump" the drug out of the cell and prevent it from harming them. Another mechanism consists of the cell ridding itself of the genes that propel it toward suicide when the drug enters the cell. In short, even if chemotherapy treatment succeeds in killing 99.9 percent of cancer cells, if only one cell survives, having acquired some characteristic that gives it resistance to the drug, that one cell can clone itself, and a new tumor composed of such resistant cells can grow, a tumor that is even more dangerous than its predecessor. As we

have said, one should not be too surprised by the cancer cell's capacity to adapt; this adaptive mechanism is the very basis of life on Earth. Even less evolved cells are often capable of finding the means to resist obstacles, as is seen in the return of diseases caused by the development of antibiotic-resistant bacteria.

STARVING A TUMOR BY BLOCKING BLOOD VESSEL FORMATION

Is there some weakness in the armor of tumor cells that might allow us to better our chances of destroying them? The answer is yes. Despite its great power, its versatility, and its enormous ability to adapt to the hostile conditions of neighboring cells, the cancer cell remains extremely dependent upon its energy needs. To grow, a tumor requires a constant supply of oxygen and nutrients. In order to procure these two necessary fuels, cancer cells have developed a very efficient strategy: as soon as an oxygen or nutrient deficiency announces itself, the cancer cells secrete chemical signals that reach the network of blood circulation in the surrounding tissues. The endothelial cells that make up these blood vessels reproduce themselves only rarely; but upon contact with these chemical signals, they emerge from their relatively dormant state and begin to reproduce at a frantic pace, forming a network of capillaries with a single reason for existence: feeding the growing tumor. In this way, the tumor gets the oxygen and the nutrients that it requires for its growth and expansion into the surrounding tissue.

This phenomenon of new blood vessel formation in response to the energy needs of tumors is called tumoral angiogenesis (from the Greek *angio*, vessel, and *genesis*, formation; **see Figure 6, p.38**). To obtain the necessary supply of food and oxygen, cancer cells trigger chemical signals, namely a protein known as VEGF (vascular endothelial growth factor), to attract the cells of a blood vessel located nearby. By binding to a receptor on the surface of the blood vessel cells, VEGF incites cells to clear a path to the tumor by dissolving the surrounding tissue and forming a sufficient number of new cells to create a new blood vessel. The tumor acquires the food it needs for growth and will continue to invade the surrounding tissue.

The importance of this process in the growth of tumors was first suggested in 1971 by Dr. Judah Folkman, a surgeon at Harvard University's medical school. Troubled and fascinated by the phenomenal number of blood vessels he had observed in tumor biopsies or in the tumors themselves, Dr. Folkman formed the hypothesis that the presence of these vessels was necessary for the tumor to grow. If one were able to block the formation of these vessels, one might succeed in stopping the progress of the

tumor, controlling, in other words, the growth of the tumor cells by blocking their access to food: a very strict diet indeed! This hypothesis led to a frantic race for the identification of drugs able to interfere with the development of tumors by blocking the formation of new blood vessels, culminating in the approval in 2004 of the first anti-angiogenic drug, Avastin™. It should be noted that the blood vessels in tumors are very different from the blood vessels in normal tissue, which are not attacked by anti-angiogenic molecules. The research carried out on angiogenesis has also allowed scientists to explore the following two concepts, which are crucial to our understanding of how we can interfere with tumor growth.

Angiogenesis and drug resistance
Until the important role played by angiogenesis was identified, it was thought that the fight against cancer could be summed up by the

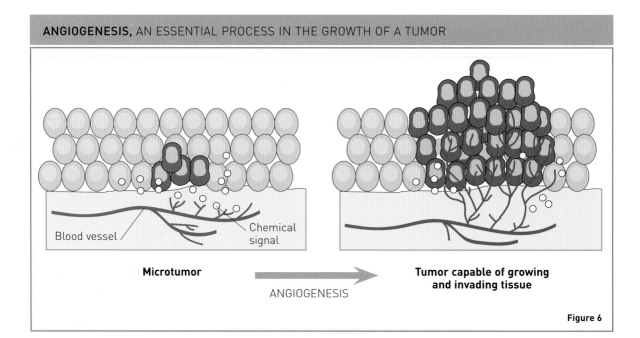

ANGIOGENESIS, AN ESSENTIAL PROCESS IN THE GROWTH OF A TUMOR

Blood vessel

Chemical signal

Microtumor

ANGIOGENESIS

Tumor capable of growing and invading tissue

Figure 6

attempt to destroy cancer cells using the strongest possible doses of medication. We now know that the development of tumors is the result of the imbalance between molecules that stimulate the growth of new blood vessels and other molecules that prevent these vessels from forming. If the balance tips in favor of the stimulators, angiogenesis and tumor growth will occur; while the victory of the inhibitor molecules, on the other hand, will restrict the growth of the tumor.

Thus there is no doubt that preventing the formation of blood vessels in tumors that have not yet acquired total independence of growth – in other words, immature tumors that are present in a latent state in the organism – could become an extremely effective strategy in preventing the development of cancer. In fact, it is now well established that in the absence of new blood vessels to supply them with food and oxygen, cancerous tumors are incapable of growing beyond a volume of 1 mm³, which is an insufficient size for the tumor to cause irreparable damage to nearby tissue.

Also, since the great majority of tumors depend on an adequate blood supply, blocking the formation of these new vessels can prevent development of many cancers. Even liquid tumors, such as those responsible for leukemia, require the vascularization of bone marrow and are susceptible to anti-angiogenic treatment.

Finally, by attacking the food supply sources of the tumor rather than the tumor itself, the anti-angiogenic approach lets us bypass the problem of resistance and adaptability of cancer cells. Even if tumors were able to adapt themselves to very hostile conditions, it is reasonable to assume that they cannot recover from a lack of food and oxygen, two factors that are essential to life.

The metronomic approach

The molecules directed against blood vessels are less toxic than the drugs used in chemotherapy. Thus they can be administered on a continuous basis, a strategy known as the metronomic approach by analogy with a musician's metronome. This approach is completely different from that of current chemotherapy, during which a very strong dose of medication is administered within a short period, followed by a stage of convalescence for the patient before the next cycle of treatment.

Unfortunately, it seems that the tumor is also able to recuperate between treatments while building up resistance to the treatment itself, especially if the cancer cells succeed in triggering the formation of a new network of blood vessels by angiogenesis. The creation of this network allows them to grow and pursue their invasion of host tissue. On the other hand, the continuous administration of medication (the metronomic procedure) has the effect of gradually reducing the number of cancer cells while simultaneously interfering with angiogenesis. Consequently, even if the eradication of the tumor takes more time, using a metronomic approach helps keep it in a dormant state that discourages recurrence (**see Figure 7, p.40**). The metronomic approach is particularly well suited to the prevention of cancer through diet, in which small amounts of anticancer molecules are absorbed daily into the bloodstream after the consumption of healthful foods such as fruits and vegetables.

In summary, cancer is a disease with terrible destructive potential once it reaches the progression stage. However, we can exert considerable influence over the development of cancer by continuously attacking the miniature tumors that are apparently lying dormant in our bodies, but that are really on the lookout for new opportunities that might allow them to advance to the malignant tumor stage. Blocking a tumor's food and oxygen supply by preventing the formation of new blood vessels very likely represents one of the most promising approaches yet; cancer cells are cut off at the source from nutrients needed for growth.

The prevention of cancer by angiogenesis inhibition is neither an illusion nor a dream: it is already happening. Certain common foods constitute preferred sources of anti-angiogenic compounds which, when administered daily, succeed in blocking the progression of tumors by blocking a tumor's access to food. These foods act metronomically, continuously attacking new blood vessels and thus preventing them from reaching maturity and being able to supply the tumor's needs. Thanks to the anti-angiogenic metronomic approach, cancer no longer has to be a fatal disease; it can become a chronic one, requiring constant and continuous treatment to control it. This kind of cancer prevention is achieved over and above all through diet.

COMPARING THE EFFECTS OF CHEMOTHERAPY AND METRONOMIC THERAPY

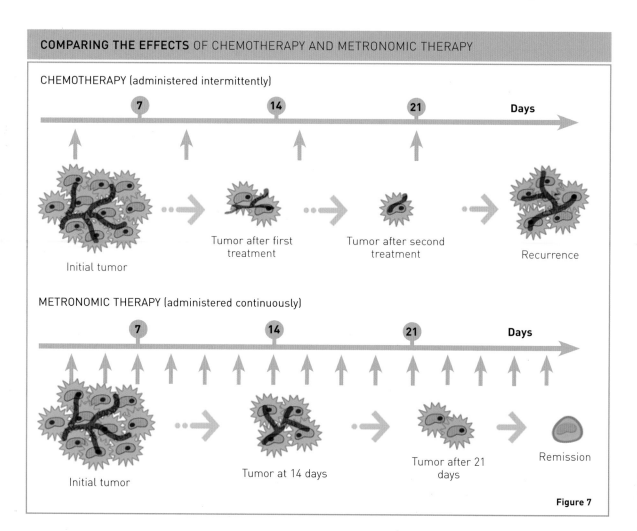

CHEMOTHERAPY (administered intermittently)

7 14 21 Days

Initial tumor

Tumor after first treatment

Tumor after second treatment

Recurrence

METRONOMIC THERAPY (administered continuously)

7 14 21 Days

Initial tumor

Tumor at 14 days

Tumor after 21 days

Remission

Figure 7

In summary

- **The cancer treatments** currently available are often stymied by the very great versatility of cancer cells, which allows them to hide from treatment and continue their growth.

- **However, tumors** have energy needs and require a network of new blood vessels, formed by angiogenesis, to grow.

- **The blockage** or the destruction of these new blood vessels is made possible by the administration of small daily doses of anti-angiogenic molecules; this also prevents the tumor from progressing.

- **Significant quantities** of some of these anti-angiogenic molecules are present in fruits and vegetables.

"Let food be thy medicine
and medicine be thy food!"

Hippocrates (460–377 BC)

Eating to Prevent Cancer

The human diet evolved over thousands of years to include the foods most beneficial to our health, but in recent times we have favored a diet that excludes many of these essential foods. Returning to a diet rich in fruits, vegetables, and other important foods is essential to preventing cancer.

The high proportion of cancers that can be attributed to the nature of the Western diet is, as we have seen, a sign of the decline in the eating habits of a society that has lost contact with the very idea of diet and perceives the act of eating only as a necessary replenishing of energy without any concern for its impact on health. Although our intention is not to try to interpret the historic and socioeconomic factors responsible for these changes, we need to stress that these thought-free eating habits, focused purely on satisfying the need to refuel, are harmful to our health. At a time when we often tend to consider progress uncritically as a synonym for benefit, we must admit that this does not apply to our diets. On the contrary, industrialization is on the verge of destroying the very foundation of our culinary traditions.

We tend to forget that everything we know today about the nutritive or toxic properties of a plant, or the use of specific foods for therapeutic reasons, is the result of a long quest by man during his entire evolutionary history to determine the value and quality of foods present in his immediate environment. What we today call "fruits" or "vegetables" are in fact the result of a process of natural selection that took place over a period of some 15 million years, during which our human ancestors constantly had to adapt to changes in their environment and become aware of new sources of food that could give them an advantage for survival. In this way, diet as we now know it is a relatively recent phenomenon: if we transposed the 15 million years of the nutritional history of humans and their ancestors onto a 365-day

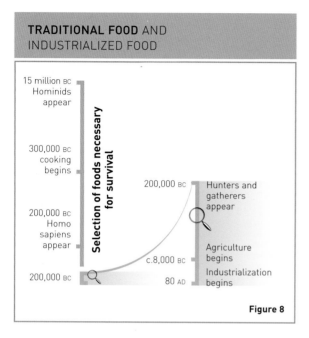

TRADITIONAL FOOD AND INDUSTRIALIZED FOOD

Selection of foods necessary for survival

15 million BC Hominids appear

300,000 BC cooking begins

200,000 BC Homo sapiens appear

200,000 BC

200,000 BC Hunters and gatherers appear

c.8,000 BC Agriculture begins

80 AD Industrialization begins

Figure 8

calendar, agriculture, which is only 8,000 years old, wouldn't have been invented until about 7 o'clock on the evening of December 31, while the even more recent industrialization of food would only have taken place three minutes before the New Year (see **Figure 8, above**).

HOW WE SELECTED OUR FOODS

The evolutionary selection process of food can be divided into three major stages. During the first stage, which we will call "toxicity study," human beings were forced to carry out multiple trial and error experiments to determine whether or not the foods available to them were edible. This was a perilous enterprise, no doubt, and one that was certainly marked by many cases of food poisoning, if not by sudden death, in the case of foods containing toxins. Of course, in many cases, the observation of other animals' eating habits proved useful and probably allowed people to avoid accidents: it is highly probable that the idea of eating oysters would

never have occurred to human beings had they not seen sea otters doing it. However, it is certain that a large number of these trial and error experiments were necessary to identify those foods that did not induce illness or cause death, and which could thus be considered non-toxic. Such knowledge was probably transmitted to the immediate family as well as to other members of the larger community. Without the communication of the results of the experiments, these efforts would have been in vain.

During the second stage of the selection process, which could be labeled the "evaluation" stage, the non-toxic foods that had made it through the first stage became dietary staples, but were still "under observation"; despite their non-toxic properties, many edible plants do not really provide any benefit to the organism, either because they do contain toxins or drugs that may in the long term affect human health, or because they are of no positive nutritious value to us. For example, eating grass is not in itself dangerous to human health, but that does not mean that grass is a good dietary choice for human beings!

The third stage, the "selection" stage, is where foods that were found to be really beneficial to health were chosen: those foods that have real nutritional value or whose consumption provides additional health benefits. Human beings, after all, do not eat solely to live; they wish that life to be as long and as agreeable as possible. This quest for longevity has led humankind to seek benefits from food that are greater than nutritional value alone; food was the only available resource that could have positive effects on health and prolong existence. Therefore it should not be surprising that the history of medicine is bound up with that of food and diet; food, for a very long time, was humanity's only medicine.

The great ancient civilizations – the Egyptian, the Indian, the Chinese, and the Greek – all recorded in minute detail their observations on the positive effects of plants and foods on health, as well as their healing virtues. The importance of good diet as a factor in maintaining health was in fact the foundation of all medical treatment until the beginning of the 20th century. Acquiring this body of knowledge about what was good, bad, or neutral to health was about more than survival; it represented a cultural heritage of inestimable value, illustrating the fundamental relationship that exists among man, diet, and nature.

If we try to imitate the ancient civilizations and write a book today about foods that are good for us, there would not be that many foods currently in fashion in our society that would deserve inclusion. This break with the past explains how, at a time when medical science has never been more powerful, we are witnessing the emergence of a host of diseases, such as colon cancer, that were rare only a century ago. However, it is still possible for us to learn from the thousand-year-old wisdom that comes from close observation of nature. Using this knowledge in combination with modern medicine can only have extraordinarily positive repercussions on human health, and particularly on the prevention of cancer.

The importance that we accord here to the historic roots of human beings and their diet

WHAT IS FOOD?

A food is a product consumed on a regular basis by a community that has been able to observe this product's harmlessness as well as its long-term health benefits.

CANCER TREATMENT BY ENZYMATIC INHIBITION

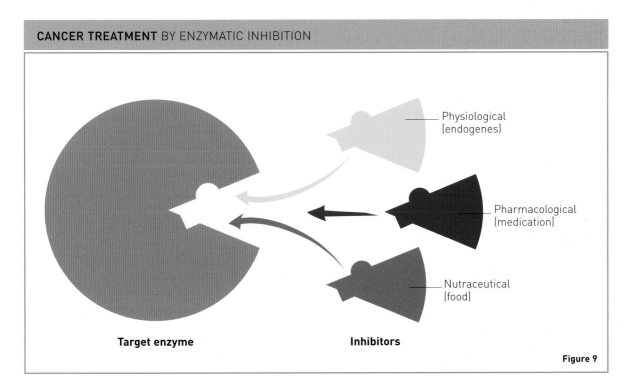

Physiological (endogenes)

Pharmacological (medication)

Nutraceutical (food)

Target enzyme   **Inhibitors**

Figure 9

does not mean that we have suddenly become nostalgic about the past! If we insist on this stressing this importance, it is because the most recent research has demonstrated that a certain number of foods selected by man over the course of his evolution possess countless molecules with anticancer potential, molecules that can really help reduce the incidence of diseases such as cancer. The current lack of interest that our society shows toward the nature of diet is not

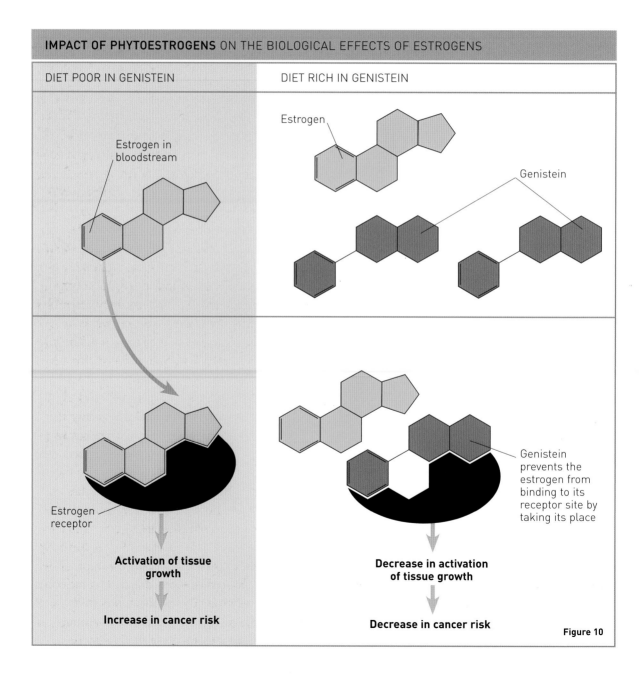

IMPACT OF PHYTOESTROGENS ON THE BIOLOGICAL EFFECTS OF ESTROGENS

DIET POOR IN GENISTEIN

DIET RICH IN GENISTEIN

Estrogen in bloodstream

Estrogen

Genistein

Estrogen receptor

Genistein prevents the estrogen from binding to its receptor site by taking its place

Activation of tissue growth

Decrease in activation of tissue growth

Increase in cancer risk

Decrease in cancer risk

Figure 10

ANTICANCER AGENTS OF DIETARY ORIGIN VERSUS THOSE OF PHARMACEUTICAL ORIGIN	
Molecules naturally occurring in food	**Pharmaceutically derived molecules**
• Known chemical structures	• Known chemical structures
• Well-defined cellular and molecular targets	• Well-defined cellular and molecular targets
• Natural	• Synthetic
• Selected over the course of evolution	• Selected in the laboratory
• No side effects	• Sometimes very pronounced side effects
• Synergy or antagonism selected over the course of evolution	• Synergy or antagonism rarely observed, due to chance

Table 4

just a break with culinary tradition but, more seriously, the banishment of an extraordinary source of powerful anticancer molecules.

FOOD, AN ABUNDANT SOURCE OF ANTICANCER AGENTS

Research carried out over the last years has shown that a large number of plants and foods included in the daily diet of certain cultures are exceptional sources of molecules with the ability to interfere with certain processes that occur in the development of cancers. These molecules would seem to act in an analogous manner to many different cancer drugs in use today.

Any class of drugs, whether they are used to fight cancer or some other disease, are always molecules capable of blocking an essential stage in the progress of a disease, acting as a kind of on-off switch that, once in the "off" position, prevents the disease from developing. In the great majority of cases, diseases such as cancer are caused by malfunctions in the function of a class of specialized proteins, the enzymes; it goes without saying that most drugs are engineered to block the function of these enzymes, to restore equilibrium, and to halt the progress of the disease. For example, if an enzyme needs to interact with a given substance in order to

advance the course of a disease, the drug of choice will often try to imitate the structure of this substance in order to block its access to the enzyme, thus reducing the latter's function (**see Figure 9, p.45**). The molecules that block enzyme activity by acting as a trap can be synthetic or natural; they can be found in foods that make up our daily diet. For example, genistein, a molecule found in large amounts in soy (**see Chapter 8, p.87**), structurally resembles a substance known as estradiol, which is a female sex hormone from the estrogen family. Genistein is known as "phytoestrogen" for this reason (**see Figure 10, opposite**).

Due to this resemblance, genistein acts as a trap for the protein, which normally recognizes the estradiol. The genistein molecule occupies the place usually taken by the hormone, reducing the impact of the biological effects caused by the estradiol, including excessive growth of tissues sensitive to this hormone, such as those of the breast. The action of genistein is comparable to that of tamoxifen, a medication that is currently prescribed for breast cancer. This example shows to what extent certain foods can contain molecules with structures and actions analogous to those of the synthetic drugs now used in the treatment of cancer, and how useful these foods may be in

THE PHARMACOLOGICAL TARGETS OF NUTRACEUTICALS

- Tumoral invasion and metastasis inhibition
- Growth factor receptor inhibition
- Inflammatory enzyme (COX-2) inhibition
- Transcription factors inhibition
- Chemotherapy medication resistance inhibition
- Blood clotting inhibition
- Antiestrogens
- Antibacterial action
- Immune system modulation
- Cellular signal cascade inhibition
- Toxicity toward cancer cells
- Cancer cell cytoskeleton perturbation
- Toxin metabolic action inhibition via Phase I (cytochrome P450)
- Toxin detoxification activation via Phase II

Table 5

the prevention of diseases such as cancer. The principal difference between the molecules present in food and those of synthetic origin has less to do with their effectiveness and more with where they come from, whether they are naturally occurring or synthetic, as well as the way they have been selected by humans. We have seen that for foods, this process requires a lengthy period of selection, while the timescale for synthetic molecules is very much reduced: this increases the difficulty of predicting or analyzing possible side effects of treatments based on synthetic molecules.

As described above, the selection of foods by humans is in some ways comparable to the evaluation of toxicity of synthetic molecules, except that this evaluation took place over thousands of years, a period that allowed for the exclusion of any kind of toxicity that might have been

associated with that food; the anticancer molecule now present in that food is free of undesirable side effects. On the other hand, despite all possible precautions, the synthetic molecule is totally foreign to the organism, with the inherent risk of causing undesirable side effects; unfortunately, this is almost always the case. Thus, even if the action mechanisms of the synthetic molecule and the molecule of dietary origin are similar, the fundamental difference between the two approaches is the absence of toxicity associated with absorbing the anticancer molecules present in fruits and vegetables (see Table 4, p.47). In fact, molecules of dietary origin have the capacity to interact with most of the receptors targeted by the drugs of synthetic origin that have been developed by the pharmaceutical industry. This illustrates once again how much a positive effect food can have on our health (see Table 5, left). Promoting a greater intake of foods rich in anticancer molecules to prevent cancer means choosing a host of new possibilities for therapeutic intervention from among a bank of compounds created by nature almost four billion years ago, via a trial–and–error process similar to that used by the pharmaceutical industry to discover and develop new drugs to treat different diseases.

PREVENTION AND THERAPY: THE SAME FIGHT

The use of molecules present in our daily diet is important because our diet may play an important role in the equilibrium of vital forces in the body, a phenomenon known as homeostasis. We can define good health in a simplified fashion by calling it a delicate equilibrium between factors that trigger illness and others that keep illness at bay, among them factors of dietary origin. If the body is lacking in specific

THE EQUILIBRIUM HYPOTHESIS BETWEEN SICKNESS AND HEALTH

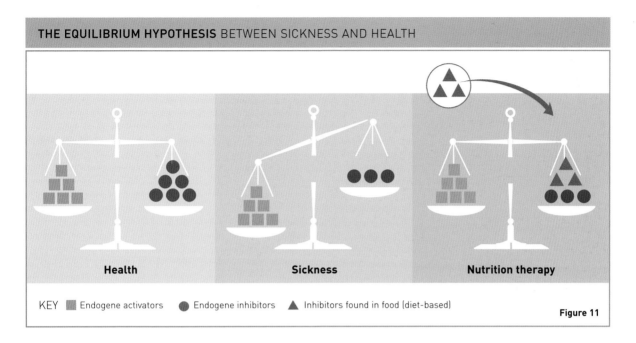

KEY   Endogene activators   ● Endogene inhibitors   ▲ Inhibitors found in food (diet-based)

Figure 11

dietary items, such as fruits and vegetables, a disequilibrium favoring the onset of illness is produced; when the body takes in the missing nutrients in the form of food, the equilibrium needed for good health is restored (**see Figure 11, above**). In this way, we can understand good health to be part of a complex phenomenon where the body's control systems can gradually benefit from compounds of dietary origin (or those of pharmaceutical origin in the case of very serious disorders) in order to maintain harmony in all of the organism's normal activities (**see Figure 12, right**).

Not only does the intake of molecules of dietary origin allow for restoring the equilibrium needed for good health, the anticancer activities associated with these molecules allow them to act as drugs that interfere with the processes involved in the development of diseases such as cancer. This cancer therapy, which we suggest calling nutrition therapy, should be seen as an important and essential addition to the means

of fighting cancer at our disposal, including the therapeutic methods that are currently used to treat cancer patients. This is as much for their capacity to act directly on the cancer cells as it is for their ability both to inhibit angiogenesis and

HOW BIOCHEMICAL REGULATORS IMPACT ON OUR HEALTH

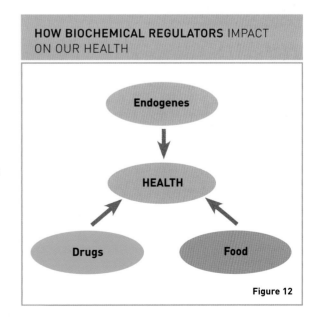

Figure 12

CANCER: A CHRONIC DISEASE

It is important to grasp that the formation of tumors is a random event that occurs relatively often over the life of an individual. Pathological studies have found microtumors that had never been clinically detected hidden in the tissues of an overwhelming number of people who died from causes other than cancer. In one study, 98 percent of individuals had small tumors present in the thyroid, 40 percent had prostate tumors, and 33 percent had breast tumors; obviously, tumors in these organs are normally clinically detected only in a far smaller percentage of the population (*see Table 6, right*).

Similarly, even though Asians in general have an incidence of prostate cancer that is several times lower than that of Westerners, an analysis of biopsies performed in a sample of both of these populations showed that the number of prostate cells on the way to acquiring cancerous properties (precancerous cells) was exactly the same in both. This indicates that lifestyle habits such as diet are determining factors that allow these microtumors to reach a clinical stage.

Why do microtumors grow?

While it is true that the tumors that form spontaneously in our bodies generally remain microscopic in size, posing no danger to health, it is also true that all too often these tumors do grow and develop into lethal endstage cancers. The development of these cancers is thought to be caused by a disturbance in the work our natural defense systems do to protect us from the angiogenesis (development of blood supply) triggered by tumors. Under normal conditions, the anti-angiogenic defenses win out over the tumors' attempts to requisition the blood supply they need for growth, and the tumors are kept to microscopic size. Individuals with Down syndrome, for example, almost never develop cancers. This protection is due to their elevated levels of endostatin, an angiogenesis inhibitor, which are in turn due to the presence of the additional chromosome 21 in these individuals. Conversely, the absence of

HIDDEN VS CLINICALLY DETECTED TUMORS

Organ	Tumors detected at autopsy (%)	Tumors detected clinically (%)
Breast (40-to 50-year old women)	33	1
Prostate (40-to 50-year old men)	40	2
Thyroid	98	0.1

Table 6

enough anti-angiogenic molecules to prevent blood vessel formation allows a tumor to acquire the blood vessel network it needs to progress.

How diet can help

The continuous presence of anti-angiogenic molecules as supplied through diet helps the body's natural defense mechanisms stop tumors at a harmless stage. Thus, even though we are constantly at risk of developing cancer, the use of anticancer molecules present in food as a therapeutic weapon constitutes an essential method of maintaining these tumors at a latent stage and keeping them from progressing to an advanced stage of lethality. In this way, we should try to think of cancer as a chronic disease, one that can be controlled on a daily basis with the help of foods rich in anticancer compounds.

stimulate the immune system (see Figure 13, below).

This method of cancer prevention is especially important insofar as we are constantly at risk for developing tumors and the use of anticancer compounds derived from food lets us stop these tumors at a latent stage (see Figure 12, p.49). Another factor that makes clear the importance of preventive therapy for cancer through diet is the existence of great differences in the genes of individuals. All human beings possess almost the same genes (if we didn't, we wouldn't belong to the same species), but there exist nonetheless many possible variations in these genes, variations that are responsible for the distinct characteristics of each individual.

These differences are not only responsible for the marked physical differences that exist among individuals, but also touch other genes, which, if inactivated, may render certain individuals less capable of defending themselves against different aggressions, such as those triggered by carcinogenic substances.

Even though only a small percentage of cancers may be said to be genetically transmissible, many genetic factors are indeed responsible for rendering certain individuals much more susceptible to developing cancer after having been exposed to known carcinogens. These people must defend themselves even more vigorously by consuming anticancer molecules. This concept was illustrated in superb fashion by the results of a study conducted in Shanghai, where individuals deficient in two important enzymes that act to eliminate toxic aggressors were found to be three times more at risk of developing lung cancer if their diet did not

THE BASIC CONCEPT OF NUTRITION THERAPY

The natural inhibitors contained in foods can compensate for genetic bad luck or poor lifestyle choices related to diet.

contain cruciferous vegetables. Conversely, other individuals who showed the same mutations but ate a diet rich in these vegetables had a reduced risk of developing cancer compared to the general population. These observations show to what extent diet can lessen the impact of genetic disorders in certain individuals who would otherwise have an increased risk of developing cancer.

It's worth repeating: fighting the development of cancer through diet means using the anticancer molecules present in certain foods as weapons in order to create an environment hostile to tumors, subjecting these tumoral microfoci to daily bombardment and preventing them from growing, as chemotherapy does. We have to see the body as a battlefield hosting an

NUTRITION THERAPY: A COMPLEMENTARY APPROACH IN THE TREATMENT OF CANCER

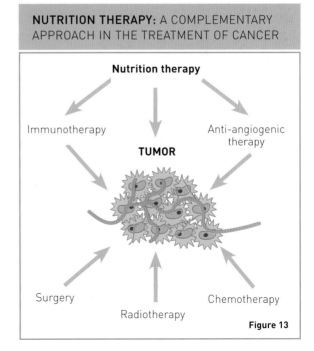

Figure 13

THE PREVENTION OF CANCER THROUGH DIET

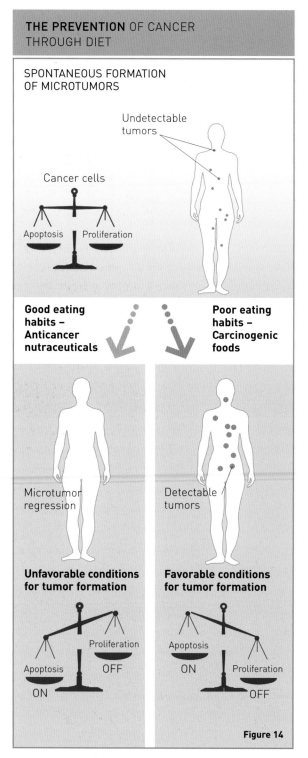

SPONTANEOUS FORMATION OF MICROTUMORS

Undetectable tumors

Cancer cells

Apoptosis | Proliferation

Good eating habits – Anticancer nutraceuticals

Poor eating habits – Carcinogenic foods

Microtumor regression

Detectable tumors

Unfavorable conditions for tumor formation

Proliferation
OFF
Apoptosis
ON

Favorable conditions for tumor formation

Apoptosis
ON
Proliferation
OFF

Figure 14

GROWTH INHIBITION BY VEGETABLE EXTRACTS OF CELLS FROM MEDULLOBLASTOMA

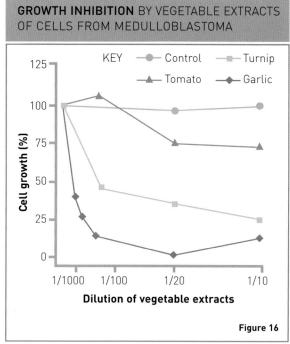

KEY — Control — Turnip — Tomato — Garlic

Cell growth (%)

Dilution of vegetable extracts

Figure 16

ongoing, never-ending struggle: mutant cells looking to develop as an autonomous entity that will degenerate into cancer, versus our defense mechanisms seeking to maintain health. A useful analogy can be made here with an on–off switch: if a diet contains mostly foods poor in nutritional quality, or if it lacks protective foods such as fruits and vegetables, latent tumors will be in an environment favorable to their growth, and thus risk turning into mature cancers (the switch is "on").

On the other hand, if diet is rich in a good variety of protective foods and only contains a quite small percentage of "dangerous" foods, the microtumors fail to grow and the risks of developing cancer are therefore much lower (the switch is at the "off" position) (**see Figure 14, left**). It is easy to see that identifying those foods containing significant amounts of anticancer molecules is something that is very important if we wish to maximize our chances of fighting the development of cancer.

NUTRITION THERAPY IN ACTION

Nutrition therapy may be compared to a kind of chemotherapy that uses the arsenal of anticancer molecules present in food to fight cancer cells that arise spontaneously.

Far from being an alternative therapy, the prevention of cancer through diet is instead a complementary tool that every individual can use to enrich his or her diet with anticancer agents of dietary origin. The regular intake of fruits and vegetables may be likened to a preventive, non-toxic version of chemotherapy that is harmless to the physiology of normal tissue and stops microtumors from attaining a stage with pathological consequences.

THE "NUTRINOME" PROJECT

Our laboratory has recently begun a new initiative – the Nutrinome Project – to attempt to establish the anticancer profile of different fruits and vegetables. This strategy aims to identify not only those fruits and vegetables that boast the greatest anticancer activity, but also the specific varieties of these foods that may contain greater amounts of anticancer agents than others.

The procedure we use requires preparing raw extracts of these fruits and vegetables, sterilizing the extracts obtained, and then using this material to determine their respective inhibiting activity on the growth of different tumors of human origin, as well as on angiogenesis, by using experimental models in the lab. For example, we can see that the addition of extracts of garlic, beets, and certain members of the

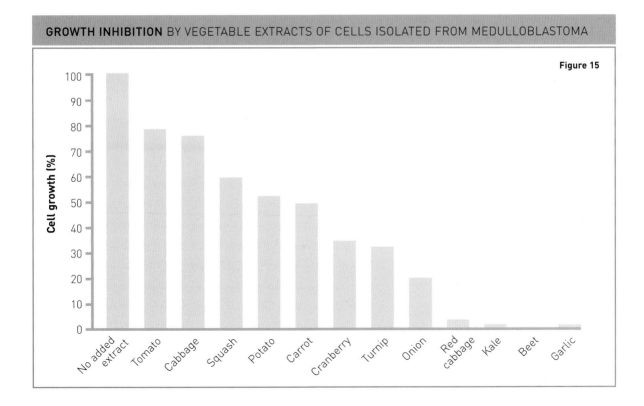

GROWTH INHIBITION BY VEGETABLE EXTRACTS OF CELLS ISOLATED FROM MEDULLOBLASTOMA

Figure 15

cabbage family, such as kale, triggers the wholesale cessation of the growth of cancer cells isolated from a medulloblastoma, which is a very aggressive type of brain tumor (**see Figure 15, p.53**). Other experiments are required to confirm to what extent these foods can be used as complements to the anticancer therapies currently available, but the results obtained up to now are very promising. Garlic, in particular, seems to be exceptionally toxic to these cancer cells. Even at a one part per thousand dilution, garlic extract still succeeds in significantly slowing the growth of cancerous cells (**see Figure 16, p.52**).

To summarize, the lowest incidence of cancer in individuals eating the most fruits and vegetables is directly related to the content of these fruits and vegetables in anticancer compounds; the presence of these compounds restricts the development of the microtumors that occur spontaneously in our tissues. A constant intake of specific anticancer substances provided by diet represents the basis of any strategy that aims to prevent the development of cancer.

▶ **In the laboratory,** research scientists are now able to observe the anticancer action of certain foods at the cellular level.

In summary

● **The foods** selected during the evolution of the human diet contain compounds that benefit human health, displaying anticancer properties similar to those of man-made drugs.

● **Including these compounds** in our daily diet creates conditions that prevent the development of the tumoral microfoci generated in the body over a lifetime. Nutrition therapy is an example of the kind of metronomic therapy that allows small doses of natural anticancer agents to be consumed daily.

● **Preventing cancer** through diet equals non-toxic chemotherapy, because it makes use of the anticancer molecules present in food. These molecules fight cancer at the source, before it can reach maturity.

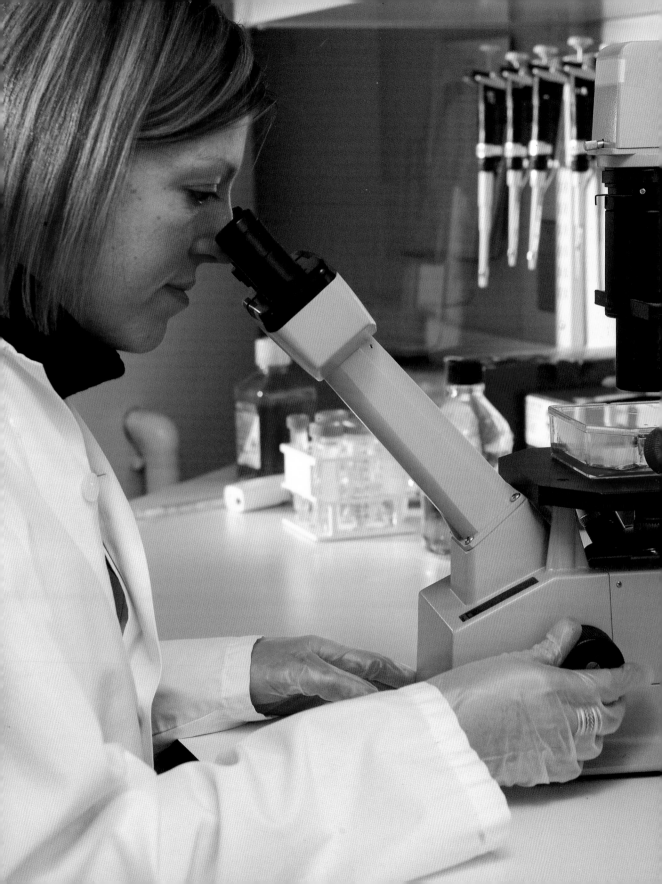

"Nature is the best physician: she heals three quarters of all diseases and never badmouths her colleagues."

Louis Pasteur (1822–1895)

Phytochemicals and Health

Among the many anticancer components that fruits and vegetables contain, phytochemicals are emerging as the most important. Laboratory studies have shown that these plant compounds have an amazing ability to inhibit cancer growth. A high daily intake of phytochemicals is vital in preventing cancer.

FRUITS AND VEGETABLES: SO MUCH MORE THAN VITAMINS!

This chapter will introduce you to the chemistry of nutraceuticals and explain how these molecules help contribute to the anticancer properties of certain foods. As discussed in the introduction, eating fruits and vegetables has long been known as a way to help reduce the risk of cancer. This allows us to suppose that these foods are an important source of anticancer molecules. If research work on the identification of these bioactive molecules has confirmed the presence of anticancer compounds in these foods, it has also allowed scientists to identify other substances present, which may play a vital role in cancer prevention.

In nutritional terms, the foods we eat are generally divided into two categories: macronutrients, which include carbohydrates, proteins, and lipids (fats); and micronutrients, generally defined as vitamins and minerals (see Figure 17, p.58). This picture, however, is incomplete. Fruits and vegetables contain appreciable quantities of compounds that do not fit into these categories. These compounds belong to another class of molecules: they are called phytochemicals, from the Greek *phyto*, "plant". Phytochemicals are the molecules responsible for the color and organoleptic properties (properties affecting the organs and the senses) that are specific not only to fruits and vegetables, but also to different beverages and spices that are often closely associated with certain ethnic culinary traditions.

For example, the brilliant red color of the raspberry, the very characteristic smell of garlic, and the strong astringent sensation we feel when we sip cocoa or tea are all properties that are directly related to the presence of different phytochemical compounds in these foods. Such compounds are present in abundance: a balanced diet containing a selection of fruits, vegetables, and beverages such as tea or red wine contains about 1 to 2 grams of phytochemical compounds. This amount corresponds to the daily ingestion of a cocktail of some 5,000 to 10,000 different phytochemicals! Far from being negligible, the phytochemical content of fruits and vegetables is without a doubt an essential attribute of these foods.

Until recently, vitamins, minerals, and fiber were considered the only substances responsible for the beneficial effects of fruits and vegetables in the prevention of chronic diseases such as cancer. However, results obtained in the last few years have cast these conclusions into doubt. It now seems more and more probable that the protection against cancer that is offered by fruits and vegetables is due mostly to their phytochemical content.

No clinical study has ever shown that massive doses of vitamin supplements can help bring about any sort of preventive effect against cancer and other chronic diseases. The results of numerous studies carried out on this field have pointed instead in exactly the opposite direction: there is an increase in the risk of death associated with taking high doses of vitamin supplements. For example, two studies done on the effect of high supplemental doses of vitamin A or betacarotene (the molecule that synthesizes vitamin A in our bodies) on the risk developing lung cancer for smokers showed that the daily absorption of this vitamin does not reduce their

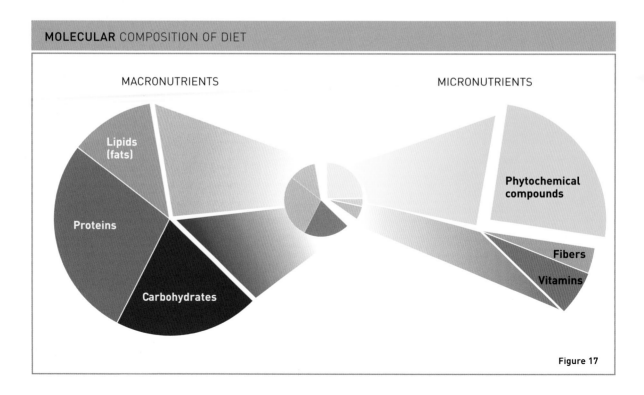

MOLECULAR COMPOSITION OF DIET

MACRONUTRIENTS

MICRONUTRIENTS

Lipids (fats)

Proteins

Carbohydrates

Phytochemical compounds

Fibers

Vitamins

Figure 17

mortality rate due to cancer. On the contrary, the risk actually increased (one study showed 28 percent more cancers and 17 percent more deaths in the subjects who received the vitamin supplement). The negative effect of supplements containing high doses of vitamins has also been observed in non-smokers.

Another recent study showed that high doses of vitamin supplements have very little or no effect on the development of cancers of the gastrointestinal tract (colorectal, liver, pancreatic, and stomach cancers); in fact, the only effect observed was a slight increase in mortality rates. Even more disturbingly, according to another study, taking 400 IU per day of supplemental vitamin E also causes a slight increase in overall mortality rates.

If you find it difficult to obtain recommended daily allowances of vitamins without taking supplements, you should take steps to reduce the doses contained in these tablets as much as possible. Tellingly, one of the only results that suggested a preventive effect of vitamin supplements in the fight against cancer was obtained in the course of a study that used vitamin concentrations comparable to those naturally occurring in foods.

THE PHYTOCHEMICAL COCKTAIL: AN ARSENAL OF ANTICANCER MOLECULES

Phytochemical compounds are molecules that allow plants to defend themselves against infection and damage caused by microorganisms, insects, or other predators. Plants cannot flee their attackers and have consequently had to develop advanced defense systems to counter the harmful effects of aggressors present in their environment. The phytochemicals produced by plants have antibacterial, antifungal, and insecticidal properties; they repair the damage caused by aggressors and allow the plant to survive in hostile conditions. For example, as we will see in Chapter 8, when grapes on the vine are attacked by certain microorganisms, the plant secretes a large quantity of a substance that acts as a fungicide and counteracts the negative effects of the parasites. Because phytochemical production occurs in direct proportion to the stress to which the plant is exposed, we might guess that plants cultivated naturally, without the use of synthetic pesticides, are more susceptible to attack and thus contain greater quantities of self-defense molecules.

The protective role of these different phytochemical compounds is not restricted to their effects on plant health! These molecules also play a very important part in the behavior of our own defense systems in fighting cancer.

Studies focusing on compounds isolated from these foods have shown that a large number of them interfere with the sequence of events that trigger the birth of a tumor. These substances could therefore represent the greatest weapon at our disposal in fighting the spread of cancer.

All plants contain a number of phytochemical compounds in variable quantities (see Table 7, p.60). It is this phytochemical content, in fact, that is responsible for the organoleptic properties that are so characteristic of these foods (bitterness, astringency, smell...). The lack of enthusiasm many people experience when face to face with a plate of vegetables is related to these organoleptic properties. While the familiar taste of fats and sugars is immediately recognized by our brain as synonymous with a quick and efficient energy boost, the bitter and astringent qualities of certain plants are interpreted as a kind of potential aggression that might be harmful to our health! Fortunately, these reflexes are controlled by the primitive brain and have gradually been worn down by evolution; human beings have consequently been able to identify an ever-growing number of plant species that may actively contribute to maintaining good health. It is often very easy to determine the principal phytochemical associated with a given food just by the color of the food, or by its smell. For example, most brightly colored fruits are important sources of a class of molecules known as polyphenols. Over 4,000 polyphenols have been identified; they are especially abundant in such substances as red wine and green tea, as well as in plants such as grapes, apples, onions, and wild berries. They are also found in several herbs and spices, as well as in vegetables and nuts. Other classes of phytochemicals are characterized by their smell: the smell of sulfur we associate with crushed garlic, for example, or with cooked cabbage is due to the presence of sulfur compounds (sulfides) in these foods, while the far more pleasant odor of citrus fruit is associated with the presence of certain compounds known as terpenes. We will discuss these different molecules in detail in later chapters, but one fact bears mentioning right away: it is the high levels of different classes of phytochemicals present in certain foods that allow them to act as agents in cancer prevention and thus be considered nutraceuticals.

WHAT MAKES A NUTRACEUTICAL?

A nutraceutical may be defined as any food (fruit, vegetable, beverage, or product of fermentation) that contains a large quantity of one or more molecules with anticancer potential. The concept of nutraceutical allows us to choose the foods that we need to include in a diet intended to prevent the onset of cancer. Although all fruits and vegetables contain phytochemicals by definition, the quantity as well as the active nature of these compounds varies greatly from one fruit to another and from one vegetable to another. All fruits and vegetables were not created equal: in terms of their value in phytochemicals active against cancer, the potato or the carrot cannot be compared to, say, broccoli or kale, any more than bananas can be compared to grapes or

PRINCIPAL GROUPS OF PHYTOCHEMICALS FOUND IN FRUITS AND VEGETABLES		
FAMILY	CLASS	SUBCLASS
Polyphenols	Flavonoids	• Anthocyanidins • Flavones • Flavanols • Flavanones • Flavonols • Isoflavones
	Phenolic acids	• Hydroxycinnamates • Hydroxybenzoates
	Non-flavonoids	• Stibenes • Coumarins • Lignans
Terpenes	Carotenoids Monoterpenes	
Sulfur compounds (sulfides)	Diallyl sulfides Isothiocyanates	
Saponins	Triterpenoids Steroids	

Table 7

cranberries. Important differences exist in the levels of active compounds present in fruits and vegetables; in some cases, a particular phytochemical occurs in a single food only. This idea is very important when one attempts to explain the anticancer properties of fruits and vegetables. Curiously, many of the phytochemicals showing the highest levels of cancer prevention activity are present only in a few very specific foods (**see Figure 18, p.62**). The isoflavones in soybeans, the resveratrol present in grapes, the curcumin in turmeric, the isothiocyanates and indoles of broccoli, and the catechols in green tea are all anticancer molecules occurring naturally in very select groups of foods. In other words, if it is true, generally speaking, that fruits and vegetables make up a large part of a well-balanced diet, we must also take phytochemical content into account in the context of a diet that is designed to reduce the risk of developing cancer.

Similarly, we need to broaden the scope of these recommendations to include three foods containing some of the highest levels of anticancer compounds found in nature: green tea, soybeans, and turmeric. Above and beyond the clinical studies that have demonstrated the anticancer properties of the molecules associated with these foods (which will form the subject of later chapters), a striking coincidence must be recognized: people belonging to the cultures that have the lowest cancer mortality rates, and to the Asian cultures in particular, still regularly consume the green tea, soybeans, and turmeric that have long formed the traditional staple foods of their diet.

SUBSTANCES ESSENTIAL TO LIFE

- Water
- Amino acids (9)
- Fatty acids (2)
- Vitamins (13)
- Minerals (13)
- Phytochemicals (10,000)

This implies that important changes are needed in our Western diet. Eating a combination of such different foods as tomatoes, cabbage, green tea, bell peppers, turmeric, soybeans, garlic, and grapes is, in a way, the equivalent of introducing thousands of years of global culinary traditions, both European and Asian, into a healthy diet. Today, this is possible for a large majority of people, thanks to easy access to foods of all kinds from everywhere around the world.

PHYTOCHEMICALS ARE MUCH, MUCH MORE THAN ANTIOXIDANTS!

Before describing the ways in which phytochemicals can be beneficial in the prevention of cancer, an important point must be made. These compounds are much more than "simple" antioxidants. It is impossible nowadays to talk about the beneficial properties of any food without someone mentioning the "antioxidant potential" of that food or its high antioxidant content. In fact, the term is used so often, and with such little meaning, by both the science press and the popular media, that one might think the only function of foods is to

---

WHAT ARE POLYPHENOLS?

- Polyphenols are the largest class of phytochemicals found in nature.

- They are the molecules responsible for the bitter and astringent properties associated with certain foods.

- Polyphenol intake varies greatly depending on diet, ranging from zero to 1 gram per day.

provide a source of antioxidants (vitamins, too, but since most vitamins also have antioxidant properties...). One might be forgiven for thinking that the antioxidant label is what makes a particular food good or bad for health. To be sure, many phytochemicals, notably polyphenols, have a chemical structure that is ideal for absorbing free radicals; such substances

SOME **NATURALLY OCCURRING** ANTICANCER PHYTOCHEMICALS

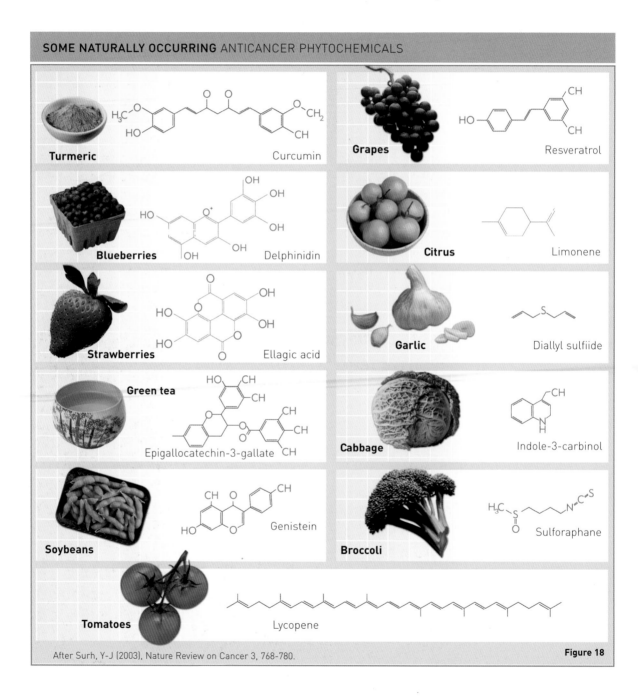

Turmeric — Curcumin

Grapes — Resveratrol

Blueberries — Delphinidin

Citrus — Limonene

Strawberries — Ellagic acid

Garlic — Diallyl sulfiide

Green tea — Epigallocatechin-3-gallate

Cabbage — Indole-3-carbinol

Soybeans — Genistein

Broccoli — Sulforaphane

Tomatoes — Lycopene

After Surh, Y-J (2003), Nature Review on Cancer 3, 768-780.

Figure 18

are much more powerful antioxidants than vitamins. A medium-sized apple, for example, which contains a relatively small amount of vitamin C (about 10 mg), boasts an antioxidant activity that is the equivalent of 2,250 mg (2.25 g) of vitamin C! In other words, there is a much greater correlation between the presence of phytochemicals such as polyphenols in fruits and vegetables and their antioxidant properties than there is between the vitamin content of fruits and vegetables and their antioxidant properties.

On the other hand, isothiocyanates, another class of compounds whose importance we will see in the following chapter, exhibit very modest antioxidant activity, despite being among the molecules most capable of inhibiting the growth of cancer. Even though antioxidant activity is a well-established property of many phytochemicals, this property is not necessarily the one responsible for the phytochemicals' biological effects. For example, two polyphenols possessing about the same antioxidant activity have very different effects on a cancer cell: one completely inhibits the activity of a key enzyme on which the other has practically no effect.

The antioxidant theory also agrees more or less well with data collected over recent decades. Even though a potato baked in its skin has over four times the antioxidant activity of broccoli, 12 times that of cauliflower, and 25 times that of

ANTIOXIDANTS: SOME NUMBERS

- An aging cell can accumulate up to 67,000 "hits" on its DNA.
- A person weighing 155 lbs (70 kg) produces up to 4 lbs (1.7 kg) of free radicals per year.
- Vitamin C makes up only 15% of a cell's antioxidant defenses.

SO WHAT ARE ANTIOXIDANTS ANYWAY?

The oxygen present in the air we breathe acts as fuel for our cells in the production of chemical energy in the form of a very important molecule, ATP (adenosine triphosphate). This combustion is not perfect; it generates considerable amounts of "waste," commonly known as "free radicals." Free radicals are harmful to cells because they attack the structure of many cell components, particularly DNA, proteins, and lipids, causing considerable damage. As a cell ages, it can accumulate more than 50,000 lesions caused by free radical "hits;" these "wounds" lead to alterations in DNA structure and contribute to tumor formation.

Antioxidants and cancer risk
To simplify matters, we can define an antioxidant as a molecule that transforms free radicals into harmless by-products, thus reducing their potential for harm. Our cells contain many substances with antioxidant activity that help protect them from free radicals. However, some people believe that these defenses are not strong enough to fight off the negative effects of a host of toxic invaders of both dietary and environmental origin: think of ionizing radiation, UV rays, and cigarette smoke. According to this theory, adding antioxidants to our diet brings in reinforcements to our cells' natural defense systems, thus helping to protect them from cancer. This theory seems both attractive and plausible, but it has recently fallen on hard times. Studies in which subjects were given supplements containing high doses of vitamins A and E produced surprising results: instead of protecting smokers from cancer, these antioxidants actually increased their risk of developing the disease.

THE ACTION PATHWAYS OF ANTICANCER AGENTS

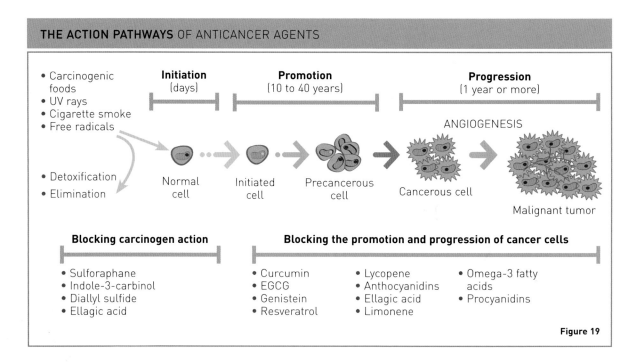

- Carcinogenic foods
- UV rays
- Cigarette smoke
- Free radicals

- Detoxification
- Elimination

Initiation
(days)

Promotion
(10 to 40 years)

Progression
(1 year or more)

ANGIOGENESIS

Normal cell

Initiated cell

Precancerous cell

Cancerous cell

Malignant tumor

Blocking carcinogen action

- Sulforaphane
- Indole-3-carbinol
- Diallyl sulfide
- Ellagic acid

Blocking the promotion and progression of cancer cells

- Curcumin
- EGCG
- Genistein
- Resveratrol

- Lycopene
- Anthocyanidins
- Ellagic acid
- Limonene

- Omega-3 fatty acids
- Procyanidins

Figure 19

a carrot, it has minimal potential as an anticancer food! It would be equally misleading to conclude that a cup of coffee, with an antioxidant content 10 times higher than that of a glass of orange juice, offers significant health benefits. It is true that antioxidant properties are a characteristic common to many edible plant foods, and they certainly do fight the harmful effects of free radicals, especially in the oxidation of blood vessel walls that is the cause of many vascular diseases. However, it is helpful to recognize the limits of this theory.

The advantage of a diet based on a daily intake of nutraceuticals is the wonderful versatility of the mode of activity of the compounds present in these foods. Far from being simple free radical neutralizers, phytochemicals can target a great number of distinct events, all of which are associated with the growth of cancer (see **Figure 19, above**). Many of these molecules even work on different levels. Some active compounds, such

as those present in garlic and cabbage, act by preventing the activation of carcinogenic substances, while others, such as polyphenols (for example, resveratrol, curcumin, genistein, or different catechols), prevent the growth of tumors either by interfering directly with tumor cells or by preventing angiogenesis.

In many respects, the processes targeted by phytochemicals are analogous to those attacked by the precisely designed drug molecules now being synthesized as anticancer treatments. This illustrates just how much foods that are rich in anticancer molecules possess an activity similar to that of sophisticated drugs. Such a combination of phytochemical compounds leaves little room for a tumor to develop; if the mutagenic activity of carcinogenic substances is eliminated right away, and the growth of those microscopic tumors that have managed to develop is controlled, these compounds succeed in keeping the tumor at a primitive stage that is not harmful to the body.

In summary

- **Edible plants** (fruits and vegetables) are not mere sources of vitamins and minerals. They also contain many thousands of phytochemical compounds that play key roles in maintaining the health of these plants.

- **Phytochemicals have** very powerful anticancer activity that targets the processes involved in the development of a tumor.

- **A diet based** on a regular intake of foods containing high levels of phytochemical compounds represents the strongest weapon currently at our disposal in the prevention of cancer.

part 2

Nutraceuticals
foods that fight cancer

- Cancer Hates Cabbage

- Garlic and Onions Ward Off Cancer

- The Benefits of Soy

- Turmeric: the Anticancer Spice

- Green Tea: Good for Soul and Body

- A Passion for Berries

- Omega-3s: the Beneficial Fats

- Tomatoes: the Prostate's Friend

- Anticancer Fruits with Zest

- In Vino Veritas

- Chocolate: a Good Obsession

I would have a man to be doing, and to prolong his life's offices as much as he can, and may death seize upon me while I am planting my cabbages.

Michel Eyquem de Montaigne, *Essays*, I, XIX (1595)

Cancer Hates Cabbage

Vegetables from the cabbage family have an almost magical ability to fight against the development of cancerous cells in the body. Although a staple of the human diet for thousands of years, many of these vegetables are no longer in favor. Eaten regularly, they are an easy way to help prevent cancer.

A Greek legend from the *Iliad* tells the story of Dionysus, the god of wine, who was welcomed less than enthusiastically on his conquering voyage to Thrace. With the help of a cattle prod, the warlike Lycurgus, king of the Edones, held back the god's army until Dionysus was forced to seek refuge in the cave of the sea nymph Thetis. Lycurgus, driven mad in his victory, began pillaging and destroying what he thought were the god's sacred vines, but which turned out to be the feet of Dryas, his own son.

Dionysus punished the king for his sacrilege by bringing a terrible drought upon Thrace, and his fury was so great that it could be appeased only by Lycurgus's death. Tortured and dismembered by the Edones, Lycurgus wept with pain before dying, and the legend states that from his tears sprang cabbages.

This is one of the very many fanciful stories associated with the humble cabbage – we have only to remember the cabbage patch, the place where babies come from! – but it nevertheless reflects the important place occupied by this vegetable in different European and Mediterranean civilizations. Cultivated at least 6,000 years ago and probably our oldest cultivated vegetable, cabbage is as ubiquitous in food history as it is in ancient and medieval literature; as the 16th-century French writer François Rabelais noted in *The Adventures of Pantagruel*, "Oh thrice and four times happy those who plant cabbages." The very cultivation of cabbage seemed to symbolize the attainment of a kind of serene wisdom.

It is therefore somewhat embarrassing to realize that nowadays the cabbage family is less than popular and does not seem to boast many passionate fans. Bland and boring for some, lacking in sophistication for others, the cabbage and its cousins are more or less cordially detested by a lot of otherwise worldly eaters. This reputation is undeserved; when harvested at the right moment and prepared well, cabbage proves to be a surprisingly delicious treat. If you belong to that group of people who cannot stand cabbage, we invite you to bear with us through this chapter. Despite all the negative publicity surrounding the cabbage family, these vegetables are heavyweights when it comes to stopping the spread of cancer.

Crucifer: the name comes from the distinctive cross shape of the flowers produced by all cruciferous vegetables, of which cabbage is the prototype. It may seem difficult to believe, but the principal species of cabbage that exist today, including broccoli, cauliflower, Brussels sprouts, kohlrabi, and kale, are all directly descended from wild cabbage (**see box, below**). In fact, it is from this plant, *Brassica oleracea*, which still grows wild along the jagged cliffs and coastlines of England, southwestern Europe, and the Mediterranean, that humans first domesticated the cabbage. They forced the hand of evolution by selecting, some 4,000 years ago, specimens with specific characteristics that agreed with the culinary tastes of the times. The Romans sought a cabbage with abundant inflorescence; they

THE CABBAGE FAMILY

Members of the cabbage family are known as crucifers, or cruciferous ("cross-bearing") vegetables, and belong to the Cruciferae family. The most commonly eaten cabbages, all descendants of the *Brassica oleracea* species, are the common green or white cabbage (*Brassica oleracea capitata*), broccoli (*Brassica oleracea italica*), cauliflower (*Brassica oleracea botrytis*), Brussels sprouts (*Brassica oleracea gemmifera*), and non-head-forming cabbages such as kale and collard greens. The edible Oriental cabbages are all descended from a different, more delicate-tasting Brassica species. Although hundreds of different varieties of cabbage existed at one time, most of them have now disappeared, probably because of commercial pressures involving crop standardization and productivity. It should be noted that the mustard plant, watercress, and radishes are also cruciferous vegetables, as are the oleaginous species of colza and its Canadian cousin, canola.

Cabbage
This category includes the many kinds of common cabbage, which are distinct in both form and color:

green cabbage, with smooth, green-white leaves; red cabbage, with purple-red leaves; and savoy cabbage, with curly, crinkled leaves, not to be confused with kale, a non-head-forming cabbage that Europeans know as crinkled cabbage.

Broccoli
Part of the all-star lineup in today's healthy diet, broccoli was for a long time a relatively little-known vegetable outside of its native lands, which are southern Italy and Greece. The word "broccoli" comes from the Latin *bracchium*, meaning "branch;" it probably owes the name to the tree-like shape of its florets. For a long time, the cultivation of broccoli was confined to the Italian peninsula; later, after the fall of the Roman Empire, broccoli spread to the area of the eastern Mediterranean basin. Broccoli appeared in France only at the beginning of the 16th century, at the marriage of Henry II to Catherine De'Medici, where it was presented as the "Italian asparagus." Similarly, it became widely known in North America only after successive waves of Italian immigrants introduced it there via their cooking; it is now one of the most popular of all the green vegetables.

wound up growing the first varieties of broccoli and, later, cauliflower. The diversification of the Brassica species is thought to have represented an important activity in ancient times; historians believe that most of the varieties of cabbage that exist today were already known to the Romans, over three centuries before Christ.

THE THERAPEUTIC VIRTUES OF CABBAGE

It appears that plants belonging to the crucifer family were cultivated chiefly for their medicinal properties in ancient times. Starting with mustard, another crucifer, which was cultivated in China more than 6,000 years ago, and continuing down to the different varieties of cabbage described by Greek and Roman botanists, many civilizations tried to cultivate plants capable of healing a host of maladies, from deafness to gastrointestinal disorders to gout. Cabbage, in particular, was prized by the Greeks and the Romans as a very medicinally important food, even taking over from garlic at one point as the favored all-purpose remedy. Praised by Pythagoras, baptized "the vegetable of a thousand virtues" by Hippocrates (460–377 BC), who recommended it in the treatment of diarrhea and dysentery, cabbage was seen in this period as a food essential to good health. This was not without good reason: Diogenes the Cynic (413–327 BC) managed to survive to the venerable

Cauliflower

Cauli-fiori to the Romans, "Syrian cabbage" to 12th-century Arabs, this cabbage cousin is probably a broccoli descendant that migrated toward the Middle East after the fall of the Roman Empire and eventually made it back to Europe. "Cauliflower is nothing but cabbage with a college education," famously wrote Mark Twain in *The Tragedy of Pudd'nhead Wilson*. Perhaps he wasn't that far wrong, if we consider the natural selection process that had to prevail for this abundantly flowered but chlorophyll-deprived cabbage (the consequence of being enveloped under a thick leaf layer) to survive into the present day.

Brussels sprouts

Sometimes the world seems divided between those who love Brussels sprouts and those who hate them. It is believed that this species of cabbage first appeared in the 13th century, but it was only later, in the early 1700s, that it began to be widely cultivated in northern Europe, near Brussels, apparently because farmers sought to maximize the available growing area to feed the ever-increasing population of that city.

This selective strategy succeeded at every level: 20 to 40 little heads may sprout from a single stalk. When their content in anticancer phytochemical compounds is considered, Brussels sprouts are in a category by themselves; if not overcooked, they become an ideal food in a dietary cancer prevention strategy.

Non-head-forming cabbages

These cabbages, of a variety known as acephala, literally "without a head," are characterized by thick, non-head-forming leaves, relatively smooth in collard greens, and very curly and frilly edged in kale. Botanists consider these cabbages, and kale in particular, to be closest in form to the first wild cabbages, and thus probably among the first to be cultivated. The father of the science of botany, the Greek Theophrastes (372–287 BC), lists in his treatises the cultivation of several species of cabbage, kale among them, a record that was later confirmed by the Roman historians Pliny and Cato the Elder. Especially popular in northern Europe, these cabbages are worth getting to know better: they are exceptional sources of iron, vitamins A and C, folic acid, and, as we shall soon see, anticancer compounds.

age of 83 while living in a miserable shack and eating little else in his diet but cabbage.

Marcus Porcius Cato, known as Cato the Elder (234–149 BC), was a powerful Roman statesman who held the most honorable and the most respected of all positions, that of censor (the magistrate charged with establishing the tax rate). He was the first person to use the term "Brassica" (from the Celtic *bresic*, or "cabbage") that today collectively describes the vegetables of this family.

Very mistrustful of the physicians of his day, who all happened to be Greek, Cato believed cabbage to be a universal remedy against sickness and a fountain of youth directly responsible for his good health and continued virility: he fathered a son at 80. Although he spent his free time absorbed in the cultivation of hundreds of medicinal plants, Cato wrote in his agricultural treatise *De agri cultura* ("On Farming", the oldest surviving prose work in Latin) that "eaten raw with vinegar, or cooked in oil or other fat, cabbage gets rid of all and heals all," from hangovers caused by overindulgence in wine to serious diseases such as cancer. He also notes that applying a crushed cabbage leaf to the breast helps heal a cancerous ulcer. Thankfully, we now have more modern methods of treating breast cancer, but the reputation of cabbage as a hangover cure has survived into the present day – a bottled salt cabbage drink that recently appeared on the market in Russia is touted as a surefire cure for the painful symptoms experienced on the morning after.

THE ANTICANCER EFFECTS OF CRUCIFEROUS VEGETABLES

Studies recently carried out indicate that the substances contained in cruciferous vegetables are among those most responsible for the anticancer properties linked to a diet rich in fruits and vegetables. For example, in a study that analyzed 252 cases of bladder cancers that developed in a population of 47,909 health professionals over a ten-year period, eating five or more weekly servings of cruciferous vegetables, particularly broccoli and cabbage, was associated with half the risk of developing this cancer as compared to individuals consuming one or fewer servings of these vegetables each week.

The same effect was observed for breast cancer. Chinese women consuming the greatest quantities of cruciferous vegetables saw their risk of developing breast cancer cut in half in comparison to women who consumed smaller quantities; this finding held true independently of the amount of soy also consumed. Similarly, a study carried out on 5,000 Swedish women suggests that eating one or two daily servings of crucifers is linked to a 40 percent drop in the risk of developing breast cancer.

Without going into all of the studies indicating that crucifers present a real chemopreventive effect, we can mention that eating these vegetables has also been associated with a decrease in the risk of many other cancers, including lung cancers, gastrointestinal cancers such as stomach and colorectal cancers, and prostate cancers. Indeed, three or more weekly servings of cruciferous vegetables have proven to be even more effective than tomatoes at preventing the onset of prostate cancer, and current research suggests that tomatoes are among our strongest allies in that particular struggle (**see Chapter 13, p.133**). If the amount of fruits and vegetables in our diet plays a key role in the prevention of cancer, these results indicate that certain types of vegetables, and especially crucifers, are of critical importance in fighting the spread of the disease.

Such observations take on even greater relevance in the context of the Western diet, and particularly the North American diet, in which potatoes count for almost half of all fruits and vegetables consumed and the presence of cruciferous vegetables remains modest at best.

PHYTOCHEMICAL COMPOUNDS IN VEGETABLES OF THE CABBAGE FAMILY

The spectacular decrease in the risk of developing different cancers seen in individuals with a diet rich in cruciferous vegetables suggests that these foods are an important source of phytochemical compounds. Indeed, of all edible plants, cruciferous vegetables are probably those that contain the largest variety of phytochemical compounds with anticancer activity. In addition to several polyphenols found in other foods that protect against cancer (discussed later in this book), cruciferous vegetables contain high concentrations of a group of compounds known as glucosinolates (**see Table 8, right**).

Glucosinolates

Contrary to most of the phytochemical compounds we will discuss in subsequent chapters, glucosinolate molecules do not act directly to prevent the development of cancer. Instead, they work by releasing two classes of compounds that possess extremely high anticancer activity: isothiocyanates and indoles.

Over one hundred glucosinolates exist in nature; they act as a kind of reservoir that stocks many different isothiocyanates and indoles, all boasting high anticancer potential (**see Table 9, p.74**). To illustrate how this works, let us take the following example: a person who cares about his or her health bites into a broccoli flower, a good source of glucosinolates. As this person chews on the broccoli, the plant cells

GLUCOSINOLATE CONTENT IN THE PRINCIPAL CRUCIFEROUS VEGETABLES	
Cruciferous vegetables	**Glucosinolates** (mg per 100 g)
Brussels sprouts	237
Collard greens	201
Kale	101
Watercress	95
Turnip	93
White or red cabbage	65
Broccoli	62
Cauliflower	43
Chinese white cabbage (bok choy)	54
Chinese celery cabbage (pai tsai)	21

From Br. J. Nutrition (2003) 90, 687-697.
The amounts indicated are averages obtained from all recent research values. **Table 8**

break down and the separate compartments that were present in the cells mix together.

As a consequence of this mixing, the glucosinolates contained in one cell compartment are now exposed to myrosinase, an enzyme that was present in another compartment. Myrosinase acts by breaking up parts of the glucosinolate molecules. In our particular case, chewing on the broccoli flower causes the principal isothiocyanate in this molecule, glucoraphanin, to find itself in the presence of myrosinase. The glucoraphanin is immediately converted into sulforaphane, a powerful anticancer molecule (**see Figure 20, p.75**). In other words, the anticancer molecules in cruciferous vegetables are present in a latent state in the vegetables themselves; it is only when these vegetables are actually eaten that the active anticancer compounds are released. These compounds can then fulfill the cancer-fighting functions that are discussed later in this chapter.

Because of the complex nature of this mechanism, several factors must be considered in order to maximize the active isothiocyanate and indole content in cruciferous vegetables. First, it is important to note that glucosinolates are very soluble in water: cooking a cruciferous vegetable for ten minutes in a large volume of boiling water reduces by half the quantity of glucosinolates present in the vegetable; this is a cooking method best avoided. Second, myrosinase activity is very sensitive to heat; a prolonged cooking time, whether or not it involves boiling the vegetable, also substantially reduces the amount of isothiocyanates that can be released once the vegetable is eaten. Some studies suggest that another myrosinase, one that occurs in normal intestinal flora, may act to compensate for the enzyme disactivation due to heat and increase the quantity of isothiocyanates that can be absorbed, but the role of this intestinal myrosinase is still unclear. Cruciferous vegetables should therefore be cooked as little as possible, in a minimum of liquid, to reduce the loss of myrosinase activity and glucosinolates caused by soaking the vegetable in water.

Rapid cooking techniques, such as steaming or stir-frying in a wok, are simple and effective ways of maximizing the quantity of anticancer molecules delivered by cruciferous vegetables; as a bonus, these cooking methods often make these vegetables more attractive and better-tasting. Frozen vegetables are subjected to a high-temperature blanching process that reduces their glucosinolate content as well as subsequent myrosinase activity; as a source of anticancer

CRUCIFEROUS VEGETABLES AND ISOTHIOCYANATES	
VEGETABLES	PRINCIPAL ISOTHIOCYANATES
Cabbage	Allyl isothiocyanate
	3-methylsulfinylpropyl isothiocyanate
	4-methylsulfinylbutyl isothiocyanate
	3-methylthiopropyl isothiocyanate
	4-methylthiobutyl isothiocyanate
	2-phenylethyl isothiocyanate
	Benzyl isothiocyanate
Broccoli	Sulforaphane
	3-methylsulfinylpropyl isothiocyanate
	3-butenyl isothiocyanate
	Allyl isothiocyanate
	4-methylsulfinylbutyl isothiocyanate
Turnip	2-phenylethyl isothiocyanate
Watercress	2-phenylethyl isothiocyanate
Common wintercress	Benzyl isothiocyanate
Radish	4-methylthio-3-butenyl isothiocyanate

Table 9

molecules, frozen vegetables are vastly inferior to fresh ones. In order to release the active molecules successfully, chew your cruciferous vegetables thoroughly before swallowing!

Sulforaphane, the star of the isothiocyanates

The structure of isothiocyanates contains a sulfur atom, which is responsible for the characteristic smell released when cabbages and other members of the cabbage family are overcooked. Because every isothiocyanate is derived from the transformation of a different glucosinolate, the nature of the isothiocyanates associated with different cruciferous vegetables depends on the glucosinolate present in each vegetable. Some glucosinolates occur at almost equal concentration in all cruciferous vegetables, while others, and their corresponding isothiocyanates, are present in very high levels in a specific crucifer. These differences in glucosinolate content are important because certain isothiocyanates show more powerful anticancer activity than others: this is the case of the sulforaphane in broccoli.

Sulforaphane was first isolated in 1959 from whitetop, or hoary cress (*Cardaria draba*), a weed in which it occurs in very large quantities. From a nutritional point of view, however, broccoli is by far the best source of sulforaphane; one serving of the vegetable may contain up to 60 milligrams. It is also interesting to note that broccoli sprouts, of the type often sold in health food stores, may contain up to one hundred times the sulforaphane found in the mature plant – a fact that should give us the incentive to add this light and healthful ingredient to an everyday sandwich more often!

Both sulforaphane and broccoli deserve special consideration in the context of any strategy aimed at preventing cancer through diet. This interest is justified by results obtained over the last decade indicating that sulforaphane greatly accelerates the body's ability to flush out toxic substances linked to the development of cancer. Far from being an isolated phenomenon, the increase in detoxifying ability due to sulforaphane sharply reduces the occurrence, the number, and the size of mammary tumors caused by certain carcinogenic substances in rats or mice. As we have seen, epidemiological studies suggest that this anticancer effect could also apply in humans.

Sulforaphane also seems capable of acting directly at the level of the cancerous cells and bringing about their demise by triggering apoptosis. In a series of studies that tested the ability of different substances derived from food to destroy cells isolated from an infantile brain tumor, or medulloblastoma, we observed that sulforaphane was the only molecule to exhibit such activity. Sulforaphane's cancer–destroying properties were also observed for other types of tumors, such as those of the colon and the prostate, as well as in the case of acute

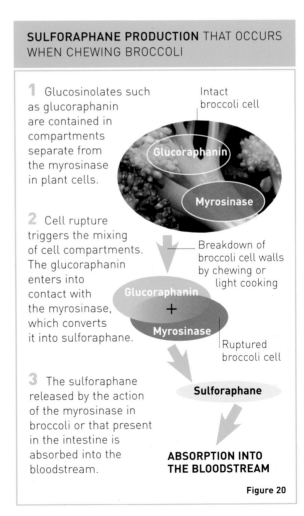

SULFORAPHANE PRODUCTION THAT OCCURS WHEN CHEWING BROCCOLI

1 Glucosinolates such as glucoraphanin are contained in compartments separate from the myrosinase in plant cells.

Intact broccoli cell

Glucoraphanin

Myrosinase

2 Cell rupture triggers the mixing of cell compartments. The glucoraphanin enters into contact with the myrosinase, which converts it into sulforaphane.

Breakdown of broccoli cell walls by chewing or light cooking

Glucoraphanin + Myrosinase

Ruptured broccoli cell

3 The sulforaphane released by the action of the myrosinase in broccoli or that present in the intestine is absorbed into the bloodstream.

Sulforaphane

ABSORPTION INTO THE BLOODSTREAM

Figure 20

lymphoblastic leukemia (ALL); this suggests that the direct action of the molecule on tumor cells is part of its arsenal of anticancer behavior.

Sulforaphane also boasts antibiotic and bactericidal properties, notably against *Helicobacter pylori*, the bacteria responsible for gastric ulcers. This activity does not at first glance seem related to cancer; it may, however, play a very important role in protecting against stomach cancer. Scientists now believe that infection by *H. pylori*, combined with the ensuing ulcers, considerably increases the risk of stomach cancer (by a factor of three to six times). Eating broccoli would allow the sulforaphane to come into direct contact with *H. pylori* bacteria in the stomach and thus prevent the onset of disease at the source. These properties make sulforaphane the isothiocyanate with the greatest anticancer potential, and by extension broccoli one of the most important foods in the prevention of cancer through diet.

However, for all the beneficial properties associated with sulforaphane, it would be wrong to assume that eating regular helpings of broccoli is the only way we might prevent cancer. The isothiocyanates and indoles present in other cruciferous vegetables also possess anticancer properties that contribute to their protective effect on health. Among these molecules, two are worthy of special attention: phenethyl isothiocyanate (PEITC) and indole-3-carbinol (I3C).

Phenethyl isothiocyanate (PEITC)

PEITC is a molecule formed from gluconasturtiin, a glucosinolate present in large amounts in watercress and Chinese cabbage. Like sulforaphane, PEITC has been found to protect lab animals from esophageal, stomach, colon, and lung cancers caused by exposure to toxic substances. It seems more and more likely that the mechanism of PEITC's anticancer activity also involves direct action on cancerous cells. In fact, PEITC is one of the isothiocyanates exhibiting the greatest toxicity toward lab-grown cancer cells, especially those derived from leukemia and colon and prostate tumors; the effect is related to PEITC's ability to induce cell death by apoptosis. This property suggests that not only can PEITC prevent the development of tumors, but it may also play a protective role in fighting existing tumors.

Dietary sources of PEITC, such as watercress, may thus provide additional defense against the development of certain types of cancer through their effects on the action of highly carcinogenic substances. Some studies have shown that a greater intake of watercress in the diet of a group of smokers (60 grams per meal over three days) was linked to a decrease in the presence of toxic forms of NNK, a carcinogenic nitrosamine found in tobacco smoke. Since NNK is very highly carcinogenic, these results illustrate the extent to which isothiocyanates act as powerful agents that protect against tumors triggered by carcinogenic substances.

Indole-3-carbinol (I3C)

Like the isothiocyanates, I3C is produced by the hydrolysis of glucosinolates, but it belongs to a different class of molecules: its chemical structure contains no sulfur atoms and the mechanism of its anticancer activity is not the same. I3C is formed in the degradation of glucobrassicin, a glucosinolate found in most cruciferous vegetables, and especially broccoli and Brussels sprouts.

The most recent research on the chemopreventive role of I3C focuses less on its role in the detoxification of carcinogenic substances and more on its impact on estrogen metabolism and its ability to interfere with cancers dependent on estrogens, such as breast, cervical, and uterine cancers. I3C seems capable of causing modifications in the structure of estradiol that reduce the hormone's ability to promote cell growth in these tissues. Results show that the growth of cervical cells infected by the human papilloma virus HPV16 (the principal cause of cervical cancer) and therefore able to develop into cancerous cells after treatment with estrogens was stopped by the administration of I3C.

In summary, the serious efforts made by our far-off ancestors to create all those varieties of cabbage were certainly worth it when we consider the exceptional content of cruciferous vegetables in anticancer phytochemical compounds, particularly glucosinolates and their active forms, isothiocyanates and I3C. Including

these vegetables in your diet is a simple way of taking in significant quantities of these molecules, and consequently of preventing the onset of many cancers, especially lung cancer and cancers of the gastrointestinal tract. The available data on the health benefits of broccoli are particularly encouraging; a diet containing three or four weekly servings of broccoli, nothing too excessive, was shown to be sufficient to protect individuals from colon polyps, important precursors of tumors in this organ. Finally, the inhibiting action of certain compounds that are found in cruciferous vegetables on estrogens makes these vegetables essential players in the fight against breast cancer.

In summary

● **Cruciferous vegetables** contain important quantities of many anticancer compounds that slow the development of cancer by preventing carcinogenic substances from causing damage to cells.

● **Broccoli and Brussels** sprouts are exceptional sources of these anticancer molecules and should be eaten regularly.

● **Cruciferous vegetables** should be lightly cooked and thoroughly chewed when eaten in order to maximize their anticancer potential.

"We remember the fish, which we did eat in Egypt freely; the cucumbers, and the melons, and the leeks, and the onions, and the garlic."

Numbers 11:5

"Garlic is to health as scent is to the rose."

Provençal proverb

Garlic and Onions Ward Off Cancer

In folklore, garlic keeps vampires at bay, but it seems that in real life, garlic and onions have an even more important role to play – warding off cancer. This family of vegetables has long been part of the major cuisines of the world. They not only taste good, they also have a positive effect on health.

The numerous historical references to the use of garlic and its cousins of the Allium family (onions, leeks, and so forth) by ancient civilizations represent one of the best-documented examples of the role of plants in the treatment of disease and the maintenance of good health in general. Over the course of the history of the greatest civilizations, garlic was always considered as much a medicine as a food; no other family of plants has been as intrinsically bound up with the flourishing of the world's culinary and medicinal cultures.

The cultivation of garlic and onions was probably begun in Central Asia and the Middle East over 5,000 years ago. It later spread to the Mediterranean basin, and particularly to Egypt, and the Far East, where it was already in common use in China over two thousand years before Christ. The Egyptians were especially fond of these plants and attributed their own strength and endurance to garlic and onion consumption. The Greek historian Herodotus of Halicarnassus (484-425 BC) relates the discovery of inscriptions on the Great Pyramid of Cheops that describe the large sums (1,600 talents of silver) spent to feed workers meals based on garlic and onions.

Far from being a working-class food, garlic was of great importance in Egyptian rites and customs, as shown by the presence of garlic cloves among the riches of Tutankhamen's tomb (from around 1500 BC). The Codex Ebers, a medical papyrus dating from this time, lists over 20 garlic-based remedies as effective treatment for a variety of ailments, including headaches, worms, high blood pressure, and tumors.

The medicinal use of garlic was not confined to Egypt, but was common to most ancient civilizations. References to the medicinal uses of garlic were also made by Aristotle, Hippocrates, and Aristophanes, as well as by the Roman naturalist Pliny the Elder, who describes in his *Natural History* no fewer than 61 garlic-based cures. Garlic was recommended for treating infections, respiratory problems, digestive complaints, and lack of energy.

Introduced into Europe by the Romans, by the Middle Ages garlic was being used more and more often to fight the plague and other contagious diseases, and much later, in the 18th and 19th centuries, garlic was used against scurvy and asthma. It was only in 1858 that Louis Pasteur definitively demonstrated garlic's powerful antibacterial activity.

THE SULFUR COMPOUNDS IN GARLIC AND ONIONS

We can imagine the surprise of the human beings who first bit into an onion bulb or a garlic clove; how were they to know that these odorless plants would be capable of releasing such flavor and aroma?

This difference in odor is explained by the chemical changes that occur in the bulbs of the members of the Allium family when the bulb is crushed. It is similar to what happens when cruciferous vegetables are chewed. The characteristic taste and odor of the different species of Allium are due to their high content of several sulfur-containing phytochemical compounds, molecules whose chemical structure includes an atom of sulfur. We can describe the reactions that occur in that little clove of garlic

THE PRINCIPAL MEMBERS OF THE ALLIUM FAMILY

Garlic
Uncontestably the world's most commonly used condiment, garlic (*Allium sativa*) is an essential ingredient in most culinary traditions. The Chinese word for garlic, *suan*, is represented by a single character, implying that it was in widespread use from the beginning of the evolution of the language. Used from ancient times to treat animal bites, such as snake bites, garlic eventually acquired a legendary reputation as one of the surest aids in warding off vampires. The legend loses some of its luster when we realize that the anticoagulant properties that are also associated with garlic should attract vampires rather than scare them away!

Onions
Native to Eurasia, the *Allium cepa* bulb is now cultivated and eaten around the world as a condiment and vegetable. Essential to Egyptian culture, which held it to be possessed of strength and power, a symbol of intelligence in ancient China, and the European vegetable of choice during the Middle Ages, the onion has long occupied an honored place in human diet and tradition. From a phytochemical point of view, the onion is a major source of the flavonoid quercetin, containing up to 50 milligrams per 100 grams. The molecule responsible for the onion's lachrymal properties, propanethial S-oxide, is released by breaking or tearing the bulb, but since this substance is very soluble in water, it can easily be eliminated by rinsing the peeled bulb under running water.

Leeks
Of a more subtle flavor than its cousins, the leek (*Allium porrum*) is originally from the Mediterranean region, or more probably the Middle East. The leek has been a well-known vegetable for a very long time, and many anecdotes enliven its history. For some reason, it was believed to be responsible for vocal prowess; Aristotle, for example, was convinced

that you may be preparing to crush before adding it to a simmering pot on the stove. For the entire time that garlic has been stocked awaiting its moment in the kitchen, the bulbs have been storing and accumulating a compound called alliin. When the clove is crushed, chopped, or chewed, the cell walls of the bulb break, releasing the enzyme alliinase, which enters into contact with the alliin and converts it rapidly into allicin. Allicin is the real culprit: it is a very strong-smelling molecule that is directly responsible for the strong odor released by the bulb when crushed. It is an abundantly-occurring molecule (up to 5 milligrams per gram of garlic), but an unstable one; its breakdown into several complex sulfur compounds is almost instantaneous (see Figure 21, p.82).

By now most people have heard of allicin, thanks to the makers of garlic supplements who base their claims of product performance on high allicin content. Without necessarily being fraudulent, this advertising is not quite accurate, since these supplements contain not the unstable allicin, but alliin. It would be more exact to refer to the potential of these supplements to trigger the release of allicin, a potential that is directly related to the preservation of the enzymatic activity of the allinase also present in the supplements. Tests carried out by an independent American laboratory have shown that the amount of allicin released by consuming supplements can vary from 0.4 to 6.5 milligrams, depending on the manufacturer. The simplest way of knowing exactly how much allicin you are ingesting is by eating fresh garlic.

that the piercing cry of the partridge was related to the bird's diet, which was rich in leeks. This theory seduced the Roman emperor Nero, who ate leeks in such large amounts in hopes of developing a crystalline voice that he was known as the "porrophage" (from the Latin *porrum*, or leek) emperor! We should also mention that the leek is the national emblem of Wales, in honor of a memorable battle fought by the Welsh against the pagan Saxons around 640 AD. Saint David supposedly counselled King Cadwallader of Wales to identify his men by putting leeks in their battle helmets. The Welsh soundly defeated the Saxons and their victory is celebrated every first of March, St. David's Day, by wearing a leek and eating cawl, a traditional soup containing leeks.

Shallots
The Latin name for the shallot (*Allium ascalonicum*) refers to the plant's original home, Ascalon (Ashkelon), an ancient Palestinian town on the Mediterranean coast. Twelfth-century Crusaders returning from the Holy Land probably introduced the shallot into Europe, where it found a home base of sorts in France. France, and especially the region of Brittany, is the now major exporter of shallots. Shallots look much more like garlic than onions; they have a bulb formed of several cloves, each covered by a thin outer layer. In North America, the term "shallot" is often erroneously used to designate green onions, which are essentially immature onions.

Chives
The chive (*Allium schoenoprasum*) owes its name to the Latin *cepula*, or "little onion." Of probable Asian and European origin, chives were used in China at least two thousand years ago to add a distinctive perfume to a variety of dishes as well as to treat bleeding and poisoning. It was on his return to Europe that Marco Polo brought back knowledge of the properties of chives.

Very similar reactions occur when an onion is chopped. The difference in smell is due essentially to the presence of slightly different molecules in the onion. Chopping an onion will not release allicin and its related compounds, but another molecule very irritating to the eyes.

THE ANTICANCER PROPERTIES OF GARLIC

The data available on the anticancer potential of the garlic family suggest that these vegetables may play an important role in the prevention of cancers of the digestive system, especially esophageal, stomach, and colon cancers.

The first indications of a possible preventive role for garlic in the case of stomach cancer came from studies conducted in northeast China's Yangzhong province, where this type of cancer is especially prevalent. An analysis of the dietary habits of this region showed that individuals who consumed relatively small amounts of garlic and onions had a three times higher risk of developing stomach cancer than those whose consumption was greater. Similar results were obtained in Italy by comparing the dietary habits of residents of the north, where garlic is little used, with those of the south, where it is used in abundance. Eating the vegetables of the Allium family often and in generous quantities was found to considerably reduce the incidence of stomach cancer.

Garlic's relatives fight cancer too

It is now thought that vegetables belonging to the garlic family may help prevent other types of cancers, namely prostate cancer. In a study carried out on the inhabitants of Shanghai, individuals with a daily consumption of over 10 grams of Allium family vegetables were discovered to have half as many cancers as those who consumed less than two grams

per day. This protective effect seems much more pronounced for garlic than it is for other members of the family. In the case of breast cancer, current data does not yet allow us to precisely establish a possible protective role for garlic: a Dutch study suggests that although onion consumption was linked to a strong decrease in the incidence of stomach cancer, it did not have any impact on the risk of developing breast cancer. However, since the average Dutch diet contains high levels of fat (one of the highest in the world), and high fat consumption has been strongly linked to the onset of breast cancer, it is reasonable to ask if this particular type of diet might not be responsible for these results.

With respect to this case, it is interesting to note that French scientists have found evidence that eating garlic and onions is indeed linked to

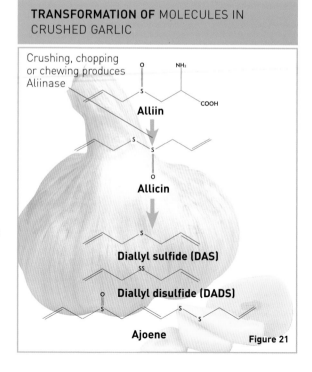

TRANSFORMATION OF MOLECULES IN CRUSHED GARLIC

Crushing, chopping or chewing produces Aliinase

Aliin

Allicin

Diallyl sulfide (DAS)

Diallyl disulfide (DADS)

Ajoene

Figure 21

a reduced incidence of breast cancer in the women of Lorraine, in northeastern France.

Current data show that the amounts of vegetables of the Allium family now consumed by certain Western populations fall far short of the amounts associated with a decrease in the risk of prostate and breast cancer. For example, only 15 percent of British men eat six grams of garlic, or about two cloves, per week; barely 20 percent of Americans eat more than two grams per week. Given the high risk these groups run of developing prostate cancer and breast cancer respectively, it is probable that garlic consumption plays a key role in the difference in cancer incidence between East and West.

These disparities illustrate the importance of considering all dietary and nutritional factors when we try to determine the impact of diet on the development of cancer, and avoid building a particular food up as heroic without taking into account the contribution of other foods.

Even though many scientists have postulated that allicin is responsible for the medicinal properties of garlic, its very high chemical instability raises some doubt as to the efficiency of its absorption into the body and its activity in cells. As we mentioned earlier, it is now well known that allicin is quickly converted into a number of compounds, including ajoene, diallyl sulfide (DAS), diallyl disulfide (DADS), and a host of others. It is worth noting that these compounds possess some very interesting biological activity of their own. In total, at least twenty compounds derived from garlic have been studied and have shown anticancer activity. However, DAS and DADS, which are both fat-soluble molecules, are generally considered to be the principal compounds found in garlic that may play a role in the prevention of cancer.

In the lab, the anticancer properties of compounds present in garlic have been studied mainly in animals, in which cancers are brought on by exposure to carcinogenic substances. As a general rule, the results obtained with animals correspond to the observations made in humans; in other words, the phytochemical compounds contained in garlic and onions are able to help prevent the onset or the progression of certain types of cancers, especially stomach and esophageal cancers, with some indication of similar activity in the case of lung, breast, and colon cancers.

Which cancers does garlic fight best?

Garlic seems particularly effective in protecting against cancers caused by nitrosamines, a class of chemical compounds with very high carcinogenic potential. Nitrosamines are formed by our intestinal flora from nitrites, a class of food additives that are frequently used as preservatives, especially in pickled foods and cured meat products such as sausages, bacon, and ham. By preventing the formation of nitrosamines, potent carcinogens that interact with DNA, the phytochemical compounds in garlic reduce the risk of these compounds triggering mutations in DNA and thus causing cancer. The protective effect of garlic against nitrosamines seems very powerful; in laboratory rats, DAS is even able to neutralize the development of lung cancers caused by NNK, an extremely toxic nitrosamine created in the transformation of nicotine during tobacco combustion. The protective effect of garlic seems to be stronger than that of onions, even though onion consumption has also been associated with a lesser risk of developing stomach cancer.

Another way in which the compounds in garlic and onions may interfere with the development of cancer lies in their effect on the systems responsible for flushing foreign substances with carcinogenic potential out of the body (**see Chapter 6, p.69**). In fact, several compounds, including DAS, inhibit the enzymes responsible for the activation of carcinogens while stimulating the activity of those responsible for the elimination of these compounds. The immediate consequence of these two properties is that cells are less exposed to carcinogenic agents and thus less susceptible to the damage at the DNA level that leads to cancer. The compounds in garlic, just like those present in vegetables belonging to the cabbage family, can thus be considered front-line preventive agents, capable of blocking cancer from the outset.

Garlic's direct action on cancer cells

In addition to their action on carcinogenic substances, the compounds in garlic may also directly attack tumor cells and destroy them through apoptosis (**see Chapter 2, p.25**). In fact, the treatment of cells isolated from leukemia and cancers of the colon, breast, lung, and prostate with different compounds extracted from garlic causes very significant changes in the growth of the tumor cells while activating the process that leads to their death. The molecule with the greatest ability to cause cell death seems to be DAS, although similar effects have been observed with related compounds, such as ajoene. We have also observed that DAS may help destroy cancer cells by modifying their capacity to resist specific chemotherapy drugs.

In summary, the anticancer properties of vegetables in the garlic family seem linked chiefly to their content in sulfur-containing compounds. Nevertheless, in the case of onions, the important contribution of other classes of molecules should not be overlooked: polyphenols such as quercetin, for example, a molecule able to prevent the growth of a great number of lab-grown cancer cells and which interferes with the development of cancers in animals. In any case, taking into account the most current research findings, it is more and more certain that the compounds found in garlic and onions may act as powerful inhibitors of cancer growth by targeting at least two processes involved in tumor formation.

On one hand, these compounds may prevent the activation of carcinogenic substances by reducing their reactivity and accelerating their elimination: the two effects combine to reduce the DNA damage caused by these substances (DNA being the primary target of carcinogens). On the other hand, the molecules found in garlic and onions are also capable of slowing down the propagation of tumors by interfering with the growth processes in cancer cells, leading to cell death by apoptosis. Even if other studies are necessary to better identify the different action pathways of the molecules derived from garlic and onions, there is no doubt that garlic and the other vegetables of the Allium family deserve a place of honor in any strategy of cancer prevention through diet. Garlic has the power to ward off a lot more than evil spirits and vampires!

In summary

● **Garlic and fellow** members of the Allium family slow the development of cancer both through their protective action against the damage caused by carcinogenic substances and their ability to prevent cancer cell growth.

● **The molecules** responsible for these anticancer effects are released when the vegetables are crushed, chopped, or chewed.

● **Freshly crushed garlic** is by far the best source of anticancer compounds and should be preferred over supplements.

CH$_2$

CH$_2$ C

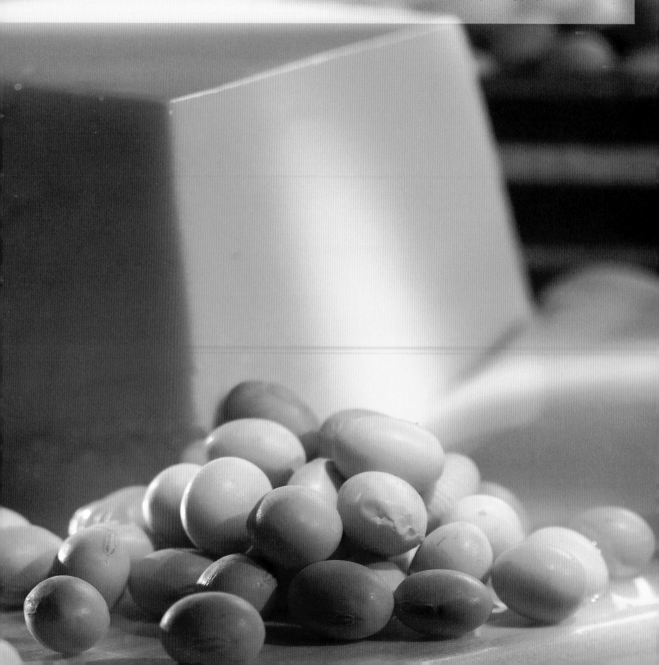

"The discovery of a new dish does more for human happiness than the discovery of a new star."

Jean Anthelme Brillat-Savarin, *The Physiology of Taste* (1825)

The Benefits of Soy

Although still relatively uncommon in the West, soy and products derived from it have formed a staple of Eastern diets for many hundreds of years. The low incidence of hormone-dependent cancers, such as breast and prostate cancer, in the East may be due to the benefits of a diet high in soy.

We do not know exactly when the cultivation of soybeans began, but it is generally accepted that their domestication developed considerably in Manchuria, in today's Chinese provinces of Liaoning, Jilin, and Heilongjiang, about three thousand years ago, during the Zhou (Chou) dynasty (1122–256 BC). At that time, soybeans were already considered one of the five sacred grains, along with barley, wheat, millet, and rice. However, according to some historians, this sacred character was mostly associated with the use of soybeans as a soil fertilizer because of their nitrogen-fixing properties: soybeans, like other legumes (such as beans, string beans, peas, and lentils), are able to absorb the nitrogen present in the air and transfer it to the soil. Legumes are industrious and efficient plants, delivering benefits to both health and ecology:

they enrich the soil in which they grow, producing highly nutritious substances over a relatively short period of time.

Soybeans were probably not included in the human diet until after the discovery of fermentation techniques during the Zhou dynasty. The first foods made from soybeans were in fact products of fermentation, such as miso and soy sauce; they were followed by the discovery of tofu preparation (**see box, pp.88–89**). In any case, it was during this period and in the centuries that followed that both soybean cultivation and soybean fermentation techniques spread through the south of China toward Korea, Japan, and other parts of Southeast Asia, where inhabitants appreciated the relative ease of soybean culture, as well as the exceptional nutritious and medicinal properties of the beans.

Even today, the consumption of soybeans and foods derived from them plays an integral part in the culinary traditions of Asian countries.

These foods may constitute a huge part of the daily life and diet of Japanese, Chinese, and Indonesian people, among others, but soybeans are pretty much unknown in the West. Only a small minority of gourmets have adopted soy and soy products. The average daily intake of soy in any form is approximately 65 grams per person in Japan, about 40 grams per person in China, and less than 1 gram per person in the West. In Europe and North America, legumes such as soybeans are too often hidden in food pyramid guides under the heading "Meat and meat substitutes," an unjust categorization when we stop to consider how rich soybeans are in proteins, essential fatty acids, vitamins, minerals, and dietary fiber. Soy is an outstanding food whose potential remains largely untapped and unexploited in our society. More's the pity; as we shall see in this chapter, since soybeans are interesting not only from a nutritional perspective, but from a cancer-fighting one as well: they are an extremely important source of anticancer phytochemical compounds.

THE MAJOR FOOD SOURCES OF SOYBEANS

Soybeans (edamame)
Edamame means "beans on the branch" in Japanese, and these beans are the snack of choice in Japan. The pods are harvested quickly to avoid an excessive hardening of the beans, and then they are lightly boiled; the beans may then be eaten directly out of the pods. In North America, frozen pods can be found in supermarkets or specialty food stores. Soybeans themselves offer what may be the most delicious way of eating soy, as well as a pleasant means of treating yourself to an excellent source of anticancer phytochemical compounds: isoflavones.

Miso
Miso is a fermented paste prepared from a mixture of soybeans, salt, and a fermenting agent, koji, generally made from rice and the *Aspergillus oryzae* fungus. The ingredients are mixed and left to ferment for a period of six months to five years. Known in Japan as early as 700 AD, miso has been one of the most important ingredients of traditional Japanese cuisine from the Muromachi period (1338-1573) onward. Historically, it was used in soup to compensate for the lack of proteins mandated by the traditional Buddhist ban on eating meat; even today, miso is still the basis of the traditional Japanese meal of ichiju issai (soup accompanied by a dish of vegetables and rice). In Japan, no less than 10.7 pounds (4.9 kilograms) of miso are consumed per person per year!

Soy sauce
Soy sauce, the major ingredient in Japanese seasoning, is certainly the most common and well-known soy-based product in the West. Soy sauce is made from soybeans fermented with the *Aspergillus sojae* fungus. Different varieties of soy sauce include shoyu sauce, a mixture of soybeans and wheat; tamari sauce, made only from soybeans; and teriyaki sauce, which contains other ingredients such as sugar and vinegar.

Dry roasted soybeans
Roasted soybeans are prepared by soaking the raw beans in water and roasting them until they turn a light brown. Similar in appearance and taste to peanuts, roasted soybeans are an excellent source of proteins and isoflavones. In Japan, roasted soybeans are often eaten every February 3rd, on Setsubun, a day of transition that is considered the last day of winter or the first day of spring according to the lunar calendar; the beans are hence known as Setsubun no mame. During Setsubun, also known as the Bean

ISOFLAVONES, AN ESSENTIAL COMPONENT OF SOY'S HEALTHFUL PROPERTIES

The principal phytochemical compounds associated with soybeans are a class of polyphenols known as isoflavones. Polyphenols are present in many other plants and vegetables, but only in soybeans do they exist in amounts large enough to be of real nutritional value.

As shown in **Table 10 on p.90**, most of the products derived from soybeans contain appreciable amounts of isoflavones; the exceptions are soy sauce (in which most of these molecules are degraded during the long fermentation process) and soya oil (often sold as "vegetable oil," containing no isoflavones). The highest concentrations of isoflavones occur in soy flour (kinako), in raw or dry roasted soybeans, and in certain fermented soy products, such as miso. Soy milk and tofu also contain significant quantities of isoflavones.

The nominal soy consumption of Western eaters may not seem all that high, but the fact is that most of us consume rather large amounts of soy proteins without knowing it. The soy-based products consumed in North America and Europe are mostly "second generation."

Scattering Festival, a member of every household puts on a demon mask and runs around the house, chased by children who pelt him or her with beans while chanting "Oni wa soto, fuku wa uchi," (Out with the devil, in with good luck!). The custom is to eat the number of beans that corresponds to your age, to ward off illness in the coming year.

Tofu
The history of tofu preparation goes back to western Han-dynasty China (220-22 BC). The early technique involved the pulverization of soybeans that had been previously soaked in water, leading to the extraction of a whitish liquid, or "milk." Tofu is traditionally obtained by the coagulation of this liquid using a natural marine compound called nigari, or alternately by magnesium chloride extracted from the nigari, calcium chloride (produced by a mineral extracted from soil), magnesium sulfate (also known as Epsom salts), or mild acids, such as lemon juice or vinegar. Tofu occupies a central place in all Asian culinary traditions; Asia's annual tofu consumption is about 4 kilograms, compared to about 100 grams in the West. Although in our culture tofu is notorious for its bland taste, its flavor can be easily modified depending on what ingredients or seasonings are added: it readily absorbs the aroma of foods with which it is cooked.

Soy milk
Contrary to popular belief, soy milk (tonyu) consumption in Asia is a relatively recent phenomenon; ironically, it was largely promoted and popularized by Harry Miller, an American Seventh Day Adventist missionary who set up the first soy milk production factories in China in 1936 and in Japan 20 years later. In China and Korea, only 5 percent of all soy consumption comes from soy milk; the percentage is even lower in Japan. Pure soy milk, after all, has a distinct, often unpleasant taste for some people, due to the presence of strong-smelling compounds produced by the enzyme lipooxygenase, which is released during the pulverization of the beans. This is why it is often sold as a flavored beverage containing quite a lot of sugar. If you wish to drink a high-quality soy milk, read the product label carefully before making a purchase: some "soy products" on the market are more artificially flavored beverages than they are true soy milk, since they are made from isolated soy proteins combined with other ingredients.

ISOFLAVONE CONTENT OF PRINCIPAL FOODS MADE FROM SOYBEANS	
Food	**Isoflavones** (mg per 100 g)
Soy flour (kinako)	199
Dry roasted soybeans (Setsubun no mame)	128
Boiled green soybeans (edamame)	55
Miso	28
Tofu	93
Soy milk (Tonyu)	9
Soya sauce (Shoyu)	1.7
Tofu dog	3
Chick peas	0.1
Soy oil	0

Source: USDA Database for Isoflavone Content of Selected Foods (2001)

Table 10

They are found primarily in industrial feed in which animal proteins have been replaced or enriched by the addition of proteins derived from soy. In this way, instead of being considered true foods, as they are in the East, soy proteins are used as minor ingredients in a host of other assorted foods, such as hamburgers, sausages, milk products, breads, pastries, and cookies.

These foods, typical of those eaten in the West, contain in general very small amounts of isoflavones, since they are made with protein concentrates that come from the industrial processing of soybeans (extraction with petroleum-based solvents, high-temperature processing, and washing with alcohol-based solutions). The soy proteins obtained through these processes have very little in common with those originally present in soybeans. As a consequence, even though the substitution of animal proteins by vegetable proteins in these foods would seem to offer some nutritional advantage (notwithstanding that the increasing use of transgenic–genetically modified soy poses important ethical and ecological problems), the addition of these substitutes does not increase the isoflavone content of food. The proteins used have been so subjected to processing before being added that any anticancer properties associated with soybeans have long since disappeared.

Why does isoflavone content matter?
The isoflavone content of foods derived from soybeans is important because these molecules have the capacity to influence a number of events associated with the uncontrolled growth of cancer cells. The principal isoflavones in soybeans are genistein and daidzein; glycitein is present in smaller quantities. An important characteristic of isoflavones is their striking resemblance, at the molecular level, to the class of female sex hormones known as estrogens; this is the reason isoflavones are often referred to as phytoestrogens (see Figure 22, opposite). Most researchers interested in the anticancer potential of soybeans believe genistein to be the primary molecule responsible for that potential, due to its ability to block the action of enzymes involved in the uncontrolled growth of tumor cells and thus stop cell growth outright.

We mentioned it earlier: in addition to their effects on the proteins involved in the growth of breast or prostate cancer cells, phytoestrogens may also act as antiestrogens, thereby decreasing cell response to these hormones.

Genistein is able to bond to an estrogen receptor site, but this affinity is weaker than that of estrogen for estrogen receptors, and does not induce as strong a response as that provoked by the hormone itself. However, the similarity in structure between genistein and estrogens allows the genistein molecule to block the site on the receptor to which the estrogen would normally attach itself, in effect reducing its access. This reduced access has the effect of decreasing overall binding to the receptor, which in turn reduces the biological effects that would occur as a result of this binding (**see Figure 10, p.46**).

Tamoxifen, the most common drug currently in use in the treatment of breast cancer, works via an analogous mechanism to that of genistein. Its affinity for the estrogen receptor is identical to that of genistein. This ability of genistein and other isoflavones to act on hormone receptors gives us great reason to hope that soybean consumption may be useful in the prevention of hormone–dependent cancers (**see box, p.92**).

THE ANTICANCER PROPERTIES OF SOYBEANS

Hormone-dependent cancers, such as breast and prostate cancers, are the primary causes of death from cancer in the West, but are rare in Asia. The omnipresence of soy and soy products in Asian diets and their quasi–absence in our own suggest that the differences observed in Western and Eastern cancer rates might be related to the ability of isoflavones, such as genistein, to reduce response to hormones, including overstimulation of cell growth in specific organs or tissues.

Isoflavones and breast cancer

Scientific literature currently cites fourteen epidemiological studies that have been carried out on the relationship between the presence of soy in women's diet and their risk of developing breast cancer. Such a relationship was suggested for the first time by the results of a study

conducted in Singapore, where premenopausal women consuming the most soy (55 grams per day or more) were found to have half the risk for developing breast cancer as those whose daily intake of soy was less than 20 grams. Other data obtained seemed to confirm the protective role played by soy in the progression of this cancer. Studies carried out in Shanghai, Japan, and the United States all showed that soy consumption was linked to a decrease in the rate of breast cancer. Recently, a large study carried out over a period of ten years on 21,852

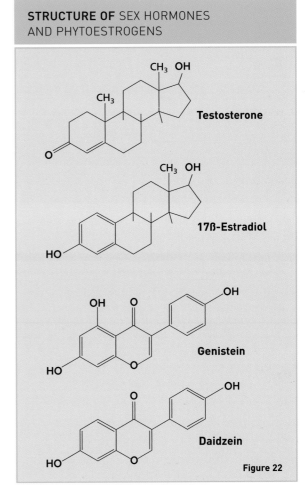

STRUCTURE OF SEX HORMONES AND PHYTOESTROGENS

Figure 22

ISOFLAVONES AND BREAST AND PROSTATE CANCER

Breast cancers and prostate cancers are hormone-dependent; that is, their growth depends to a large degree on sex hormone levels in the bloodstream. Under normal conditions, the amounts of these hormones present in the body is under strict surveillance by several control systems, which check to make sure that hormone levels do not go over a certain limit. These checks and controls are crucial because hormones such as estrogen are powerful stimulators of cell growth; excessive levels of these hormones in the bloodstream may trigger the uncontrolled cell growth that leads to cancer. It is for this reason that in the case of patients with breast cancer, for example, it is common to observe much higher estrogen levels than those in women who do not have the disease.

How is diet implicated?
The factors responsible for the elevated levels of sex hormones in people who have cancer are still not well understood, but may include aspects of diet. For example, a diet heavy in animal fat, coupled with the excess body weight associated with such a diet, represents a major risk factor in the development of hormone-dependent cancers, such as endometrial and breast cancers. Obese

women also have elevated blood insulin levels. Insulin, through a series of highly complex mechanisms, radically modifies the body's estrogen and progesterone levels. When the levels of these hormones rise significantly, an overstimulation of endometrial or breast tissue cells occurs, leading to excessive cell growth in these tissues.

Soy and prostate cancer
The part played by androgens in the development of prostate cancer is no longer in doubt. The runaway growth of the prostate seems to be almost inevitable in men of a certain age: about 30 percent of 50-year-old men have latent prostate cancer. Many factors relating to diet have been suggested as triggers that may favor the progression of prostate cancer: two examples are obesity and a diet high in animal fat. Controlling the growth of these latent tumors through the consumption of foods such as soy takes on great importance as a result. Furthermore, the protection afforded by soy against prostate cancer is not limited to its blocking effect on androgen receptors but includes its inhibiting activity toward growth factor receptors and angiogenesis (development of blood supply for tumor growth).

Japanese women showed that the daily consumption of miso soup and a daily isoflavone intake of 25 grams was linked to a strong decrease in the risk of developing breast cancer. Paradoxically, a large study carried out on a population of 111,526 teachers in California showed no correlation between soy in diet and the risk of developing breast cancer: similar results were obtained by three other studies done on smaller populations.

What should we conclude from this contradictory data? First of all, it is important to note that in several studies where soy consumption was found not to correlate with a

decreased risk factor, the isoflavone intake was very low. For example, in a study conducted on non–Asian women in San Francisco, the levels of isoflavone intake were only 3 milligrams per day for the women who consumed the greatest amounts of soy; this intake was represented mostly by soy proteins added to industrially processed foods. Barely 10 percent of these women consumed miso or tofu more than once a month, compared to an intake of three times per day for Japanese women at low risk for developing the disease! In fact, the isoflavone content in diet for the group of women in the California study with the highest soy intake

(3 milligrams per day) was half of that of the group with the smallest soy intake in the Japanese study, a group for which no protective effect was observed. It is thus likely that a certain threshold of soy intake is necessary to cause a decrease in the risk of developing breast cancer; in all studies suggesting such a protective role, a soy intake corresponding to an isoflavone content of more than 25 milligrams is associated with a marked decrease in the risk factor for breast cancer.

Secondly, it seems that a key factor that might influence the decrease in breast cancer rates is the age at which soy was introduced into diet. When studies focused on the risk of developing breast cancer by examining soy consumption in women before puberty and during adolescence, a very strong correlation was found between a decrease in breast cancer incidence and soy intake at an early age. This early soy consumption may be very important, because the protection against breast cancer that ensues continues on in life, even in women whose soy intake decreases with age.

Evidence from population studies

For example, although Japanese women emigrating to the United States see their risk of developing breast cancer rise to correspond roughly to that of American-born women, it has been clearly demonstrated that this risk decreases sharply when women emigrate at a later age. In other words, the longer these women were exposed to a diet in which soy occupied an important place, the lower their risks were of developing breast cancer, even if their diet habits had changed as adults. These observations correlate perfectly with results obtained in the laboratory that show that rats fed a diet rich in soy before puberty became more resistant to a carcinogenic compound that triggered the formation of breast tumors than did rats who were put on a soy diet only at adulthood. It would seem that soy consumption at an early age, and especially during puberty, might constitute a critical part of the anticancer effect of this food.

Isoflavones and prostate cancer

As we have seen earlier, it has become self-evident that the nature of diet is an essential factor in the alarming rates of prostate cancer in Western societies. Just as with breast cancer, Asians have prostate cancer rates that are several times lower than those of North Americans and Europeans despite having similar numbers of latent tumor clusters. This again suggests that the Asian diet contains substances that prevent these latent tumors from developing into full-blown tumors with potentially fatal outcomes.

However, unlike breast cancer, relatively few studies have focused on the role of isoflavones contained in soy in the prevention of prostate cancer. One study carried out on 8,000 Hawaiian men of Japanese descent did suggest that the consumption of rice and tofu was associated with a decrease in the risk of developing this disease. Similarly, a study conducted on 12,395 Seventh-Day Adventists living in California indicated that drinking at least one daily serving of soy milk led to a significant decrease, of about 70 percent, in the risk of prostate cancer. It would seem possible that a diet in which soy holds an important place plays an important role in the prevention of prostate cancer! These results have been strongly corroborated by studies carried out on laboratory animals.

Overall, the studies that have been conducted up to now show clearly the important role of soy in the prevention of breast cancer and prostate cancer. It appears that the great difference between the rates of these cancers in the East and in the West are for the most part attributable to profound differences in the respective traditional diet.

On one hand, a diet containing large amounts of animal fats consumed by overweight or obese persons favors the development of cancer in these persons; on the other hand, the moderate but constant and long-term consumption of foods derived from soy reduces the probability of unchecked cell growth in breast or prostate tissues. This example beautifully illustrates the concept of metronomic therapy through diet that we saw in Chapter 3: an active phytochemical compound keeps tumors in a permanently dormant state. These tumors would otherwise be engaged in a life-long struggle to reproduce and spread.

THE CONTROVERSY SURROUNDING SOY

Although a large majority of scientists, physicians, nutritionists, and others with a concern in public health agree that including soy in the diet is a positive factor for health, a certain controversy still rages around its safety for two particular groups: menopausal women and women who have or who have had breast cancer. This controversy is based on the weakly estrogenic character of isoflavones, as well as on contradictory results obtained with laboratory animals on which mammary tumors were grafted. The nature and the sheer number of conflicting facts circulated in the media makes this topic worth looking at more closely.

Soy and menopause

Menopause occurs when women age; reproductive function is lost as levels of the female sex hormones estrogen and progesterone

in the bloodstream drop sharply. Unfortunately, this normal life event is often associated with specific discomforts: intense hot flashes, the drying out of vaginal mucus, and, more importantly, an increase in the risk of cardiac diseases and a lessening of bone mass (osteoporosis). Hormone replacement therapy, or HRT, was developed to restore the missing hormones no longer being produced by the ovaries, and relieve or attenuate some of the more disagreeable symptoms that accompany hormonal decrease.

The benefits of this approach have been thrown into doubt by the results of a study showing that treatment with HRT was associated with an overall increase in risk to women's health, particularly an increase in the risk for breast cancer (which is in the order of 2.3 percent per year of treatment). Aware of these results, more and more women are refusing hormone replacement therapy. Although 40 percent of all Western women still choose to take replacement hormones to begin with, only 15 percent of them continue with the therapy over the long term.

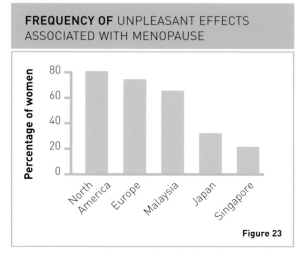

FREQUENCY OF UNPLEASANT EFFECTS ASSOCIATED WITH MENOPAUSE

Percentage of women

North America, Europe, Malaysia, Japan, Singapore

Figure 23

Without wishing to pass judgment on the benefits or risks of hormone replacement therapy, we need to emphasize the results of this study, because it is in the context of an alternative therapy that the use of foods rich in isoflavones is often envisioned. The fact is that the severity and frequency of the discomforts associated with menopause are much less pronounced in Asian women than in their Western counterparts: barely 14 percent of Chinese women and 25 percent of Japanese women report experiencing hot flashes, while 70 to 80 percent of North American and European women complain of these symptoms (see Figure 23, opposite).

As with breast cancer, the noticeable difference in soy consumption by women from these two distinct dietary traditions has once again been suggested as the determining factor in the variations observed. Such findings have spurred the inevitable appearance on the market of supplements enriched in isoflavones that are derived from soy extracts or red clover, another rich source of isoflavones.

Too much of a good thing?

The existence and popularity of these supplements is cause for some concern, since substances rich in isoflavones accelerate the development of breast cancers in laboratory mice with low estrogen levels, proportionally similar to those of menopausal women. These results seem to concur with those of the study previously discussed. Isoflavone supplements become even more worrisome when we consider the findings of another study: the administration of a mixture of soy proteins to women aged between 30 and 58 triggered an increase in several markers associated with a risk in developing breast cancer, such as the appearance of hyperplastic cells and an increase in blood estrogen levels. Overall, this data has led several researchers to suggest that menopausal women and women who have or have had breast cancer avoid eating soy.

We believe that it is important to distinguish between two very different phenomena before drawing any hasty conclusions. In the specific case of menopause, this polemic makes no sense. There is no evidence that soy is harmful to women's health, whether they are pre- or post-menopausal; we know this much from the low rates of cancer in countries where large amounts of soy are consumed. The harmful effect at issue here is the one caused by consuming prepared substances enriched in isoflavones, which have very little in common with whole foods made from soy.

Instead of gradually introducing soy into the daily diet so that quantities similar to those consumed by Asian women are eventually reached, the immediate reflex in our society is to isolate the active compounds in this food and commercialize them in the form of supplements, ideally with the highest possible concentration of isoflavones that can be promoted and expected to sell. This is at the heart of the current dilemma concerning phytoestrogens during menopause: many North American and European women now consume enormous quantities of these molecules, in amounts that have no relation to the amounts present in a traditional Asian diet. We must remember that Asians generally consume about 40 to 60 grams of whole soy per day, which corresponds to a maximum isoflavone content of 60 milligrams. In the course of a study focusing on the impact of miso soup on the risk of breast cancer, low-risk women were found to have a daily isoflavone intake of 25 milligrams; some over-the-counter supplements now available and commercialized without any government regulation may contain up to 100 milligrams per tablet! The consequences arising from the intake of such high doses of pure isoflavones cannot be accurately predicted. After all, isoflavones, like any hormones, may induce too enthusiastic a reaction from hormone-sensitive tissues when they are present at high levels.

SOY AND EXISTING BREAST CANCER

For women who now have breast cancer, or who have fought the disease and are now in remission, the situation appears to be more complex. Over 75 percent of breast cancers are diagnosed in women over the age of 50; in the vast majority of cases, these cancers are estrogen-dependent. Since the estrogen-progesterone combination increases the risk of breast cancer, some scientists have speculated that the ability of the isoflavones present in soy to interact with estrogen receptors could promote the development of mammary tumors in women whose estrogen levels are low and who may have residual or existing tumors. This hypothesis is supported by the observation that the administration of supplements enriched in isoflavones to mice with estrogen-dependent mammary tumors triggered the rampant growth of these tumors.

Evidently, a large part of this controversy arises once again from the use of substances enriched in isoflavones. In light of what we have just seen for menopause, it seems obvious that women who have breast cancer must avoid all contact with isoflavone supplements in any form. A recent study showed that although substances containing purified isoflavones did indeed cause an increase in the growth of mammary tumors already present in laboratory animals, the food itself, even with an equivalent isoflavone content, had no effect on cell growth.

These results agree with epidemiological studies showing that not only did Asian women have a much a lower incidence of breast cancer, but those stricken with the disease had higher survival rates. These results would indicate that the moderate consumption of dietary soy has no real negative impact on the further progression of breast cancer in women who already have the disease. However, another recent study conducted on laboratory animals suggests that small amounts of dietary soy cancel out the protection supplied by tamoxifen, the drug most often used to prevent the recurrence of breast cancer; this nullifyng effect leads to an increase in mammary tumors in these animals.

Although it is always difficult to extrapolate results obtained with laboratory animals to humans, it is impossible, for the moment, to predict with certainty either the positive or negative impact of soy consumption on the risk of breast cancer recurrence. As a consequence, women with breast cancer or who are in remission should consume any dietary soy in strict moderation, while favoring other foods with the potential to prevent the development of breast cancer, such as omega-3 fatty acids (**see Chapter 12, p.127**) or the glucosinolates present in vegetables belonging to the cabbage family (**see Chapter 6, p.69**).

In summary, these examples illustrate the extent to which it is preferable, on the one hand, to always consume in moderation foods containing compounds as powerful as isoflavones and, on the other hand, to avoid introducing these molecules into the body in the form of nutritional supplements, which are not representative of the nature of the whole food. Despite the controversy surrounding soy, it is important to mention that the best study on the potential health benefits of soy was conducted by Asians themselves over the last few millennia, and that the results obtained are very impressive! Soy consumption during childhood and adolescence or during menopause has never posed any risk to this huge population. We may conclude that the moderate consumption of soy, about 50–100 grams per day, corresponding to an isoflavone intake of about 25–40 milligrams, can only have a positive impact on health by reducing considerably the risk of breast and prostate cancers, which are, after all, the primary cancers afflicting Western society.

Likewise, genistein, the principal active ingredient in these foods, is not only a phytoestrogen but a molecule with the power to prevent the appearance of tumors, primarily by preventing angiogenesis, the formation of the new blood vessels that are a tumor's supply lines.

In summary

- **The great differences** in the rates of hormone-dependent cancers (breast and prostate cancers) between East and West may be due to the consumption of soy-based foods in Asian countries, especially if consumption begins before puberty.

- **Isoflavones,** the anticancer compounds present in soy, possess a chemical structure similar to that of sex hormones and may thus interfere with the development of cancers caused by high levels of these hormones in the bloodstream.

- **The key to** benefiting from the anticancer effects of soy lies in eating about 2 ounces (50 grams) per day of the whole food, such as raw or dry roasted soybeans. Supplements containing isoflavones should be avoided.

"Cookery means knowledge of Medea and of Circe and of Helen and the Queen of Sheba. It means the knowledge of all herbs and fruits and balms and spices; and all that is healing and sweet in the fields and groves, and savory in meats."

John Ruskin (1819–1900)

Turmeric: the Anticancer Spice

Used for centuries in India as a staple spice, and part of the ancient Ayurvedic tradition of medicine, turmeric seems to be able to interfere with the development of certain cancers. It deserves to be known more widely in the West – add turmeric to your spice rack and to your daily diet.

Given the ubiquity and overall pervasiveness of spices in today's kitchens, it is difficult to imagine that these substances could once have represented a commodity as precious as gold or oil. Nevertheless, for almost two thousand years, the discovery of new spices inflamed Europe, stirred up the desire of kings, and served as motivation for dangerous voyages to discover new routes that would open up the way to these riches. Without the desire for wealth and power represented by the search for spices, the explorer Vasco da Gama would not have rounded the Cape of Good Hope any more than Columbus or Jacques Cartier would have discovered the Americas.

The reasons why human beings attached such importance to spices remain mysterious. For some people, it is likely that spices were used first and foremost to mask the bland, unpleasant, or imperfectly preserved taste of certain foods, especially meats, which were conserved using large amounts of salt. For others, spices were a sort of luxury commodity reserved for the wealthy, one that allowed them to show off their fortune and social status. For example, we know that saffron was thrown in the path of the emperor Nero as he entered Rome, and ginger, cardamom, pepper, and sugar have all served at some point as legal currency due to their rarity. Spices, in other words, have long been considered symbols of both affluence and influence.

Since rarity is a prerequisite for turning an object into a valuable commodity, it is equally likely that the far-off origins of spices contributed largely to their becoming the stuff of myth and therefore, much sought-after. In fact, undertaking a voyage to discover and bring back spices became a synonym for traveling to the Orient, particularly to China and India, since the great majority of the spices with which we are familiar, such as ginger, cardamom, cinnamon, nutmeg, and saffron, come from plants that grow only in those parts of the world. Now that we know about the high levels of anticancer compounds associated with some of these spices, we can only be thankful that we have such easy access to such riches.

The word "spice" comes from the Latin word *species*, meaning "kind" or "sort", and later "spices, goods, wares" by way of the Old French *espice*. During the Middle Ages, spices were sold in specialized shops; the French word for "grocery store", *épicerie*, carries over this lost meaning. In the Middle Ages, it even became common to pay for the services of a lawyer or other professional work in pounds of peppercorns or other spices.

WHERE DOES TURMERIC COME FROM?

Turmeric is the brilliant yellow powder obtained by crushing the dried stalk of the *Curcuma longa* plant, a tropical perennial shrub belonging to the ginger family (Zingiberaceae) and found primarily in India and Indonesia. Turmeric is a sacred spice in these countries, especially in India, where it has long occupied an important place in social, cultural, and medicinal traditions. Turmeric is a staple of India's daily diet: Indians consume on average 1.5 to 2 grams per person per day and no other food discussed in this book is so specifically linked to the culture of a single country.

Although it was known in early Europe, turmeric has never really caught on as a part of Western culinary and medicinal tradition. It was appreciated chiefly for its color; the Greeks used it to dye their clothing yellow and medieval dyers mixed it with indigo to obtain a beautiful shade of green. Even today, turmeric remains a

TURMERIC

The Latin name for the turmeric plant, *Curcuma longa*, comes from the Arabic *kurkum*, meaning "saffron"; turmeric is also known as Indian saffron or, in Chinese, *jianghuang*, "yellow ginger". In an account from 1280, Marco Polo mentions the discovery of "a plant having all the properties of true saffron, the same scent and the same color, yet which is not saffron". The word "turmeric" comes from the Old French term *terre-mérite*, now obsolete, which in turn comes from the Latin *terra merita*, or "meritorious earth", probably because ground turmeric resembles valuable mineral pigments similar to ochre.

Is turmeric the same as curry?

Turmeric should not be confused with curry powder. "Curry" derives from the Tamil *kari*, a term designating any dish prepared with a spicy sauce. This word was incorrectly interpreted by British colonizers, who thought it referred to the spices themselves that were used in the preparation of such dishes. Curry is not a single spice but a spice mixture made up of about 20-30 percent turmeric, usually combined with coriander, cumin, cardamom, fenugreek, and different kinds of pepper (Cayenne, red, and black). Many versions of curry exist, with varying amounts of pepper, and this unpredictable variation can create some real heat for imprudent diners! As a bonus, a curried meal risks being a literally unforgettable experience: studies have shown that Indians have one of the world's lowest rates of Alzheimer's disease, five times lower than that of the West.

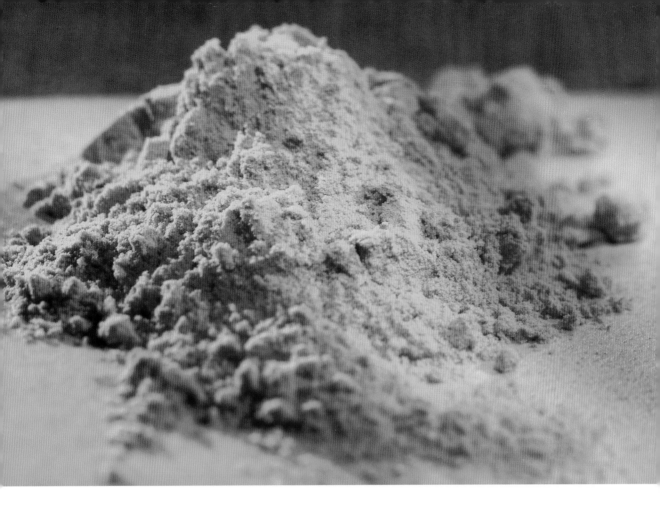

little-known spice under its own name, although it serves as the yellow food coloring in North American prepared mustard hidden under the anonymous code name "E100". Turmeric content in mustard is approximately 50 milligrams per 100 grams; a North American would need to consume the equivalent of nine pounds of mustard per day to have a turmeric intake similar to that of an Indian!

THE THERAPEUTIC PROPERTIES OF TURMERIC

Turmeric was already featured in the list of over two hundred and fifty medicinal plants mentioned in a series of medical treatises dating from 3000 BC, written in cuneiform on stone tablets, collected by King Assurbanipal (669–627 BC), and published in the mid-twentieth century

▲ **Rich** in anticancer properties, as well as in flavor and color, turmeric has long been an essential ingredient in Indian cuisines.

by the English archaeologist R.C. Thompson under the title *A Dictionary of Assyrian Botany*.

Scientists' interest in turmeric as a food perhaps capable of preventing cancer grew from our awareness of its presence in numerous past medicinal traditions. Turmeric has an honored place in the Indian Ayurvedic tradition (from *ayur*, life, and *vedic*, knowledge).

Probably humanity's oldest repository of medical knowledge (the first Ayurvedic school was founded in 800 BC), Ayurvedic medicine forms the cornerstone of the three major Asian medicines (Chinese, Tibetan, and Islamic) and is still widespread in India, where it is regarded as

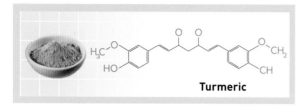

Turmeric

both a valuable and a viable alternative to Western medicine. In the Ayurvedic tradition, turmeric, considered a food with cleansing and purifying properties, is used to treat a wide variety of physical ailments, including digestive disorders, fever, infections, arthritis, and dysentery, as well as jaundice and other problems associated with the liver.

Indians are not the only people to have attributed beneficial health properties to turmeric. Chinese medicine also uses turmeric to treat liver ailments, congestion, and bleeding. Turmeric was especially popular in the Okinawa region, in the Ryukyus Islands in southern Japan, where it was known as *ucchin* and frequently used in the time of the Ryukyuan kingdom, between the 12th and 17th centuries, as a medicine, spice, and coloring agent (for the *takuan*, a marinated radish). After the invasion of these islands by the Satsuma clan in 1609, turmeric was forgotten, but it has recently resurfaced and become very popular, especially as a tea. Celebrated for their longevity (an average of 86 years for women and 77 for men) and

for the unusually high number of centenarians in their midst (34 per hundred thousand inhabitants, compared to 10 per hundred thousand in the United States), the inhabitants of Okinawa believe *ucchin* to be one of the foods contributing to their exceptional good health.

CURCUMIN AND THE ANTICANCER PROPERTIES OF TURMERIC

To our knowledge, no epidemiological study has ever explored the potential link between turmeric intake and cancer rates. Despite this, there is a certain consensus in the scientific community around the idea that turmeric may be the reason for the disparity between the rates of certain cancers in India and Western countries (**see Table 11, below**). This hypothesis is based on the fact that turmeric is almost exclusively

COMPARISON OF CANCER RATES IN INDIA AND THE UNITED STATES				
	INDIA		UNITED STATES	
	Men	**Women**	**Men**	**Women**
Cancer rates, all sites except skin	99	104	361	283
Lung	9	2	59	34
Colon/Rectum	5	3	41	31
Breast	–	19	–	91
Ovary	–	5	–	11
Endometrial	–	2	–	16
Prostate	5	–	104	–
Liver	2	2	4	2
Bladder	3	1	23	5
Kidney	1	0.5	11	6

Rates are per 100,000 population
Source: GLOBOCAN 2000. Cancer Incidence, Mortality and Prevalence Worldwide. Lyon, France: IARC Press, 2001.

Table 11

consumed in India, and there in large amounts, as well as on impressive laboratory results concerning the anticancer properties of curcumin, turmeric's primary active ingredient.

The curcuminoids are the principal compounds present in turmeric (accounting for about 5 percent of the weight of the dried stalk). They are responsible not only for turmeric's intense yellow color but also for the beneficial effects associated with eating this spice. Curcumin possesses complex pharmacological activity, including antithrombotic, hypocholesterolemic, and antioxidant properties (it is several times as potent an antioxidant as vitamin E), as well as very strong potential as an anticancer agent.

The anticancer effect of curcumin in laboratory animals has been well established by the observation that administering this molecule to mice prevents the appearance of tumors induced by different carcinogens. Studies showed that curcumin might be useful in the prevention and treatment of several different types of cancers, including stomach, intestinal, colon, skin, and liver cancers; the effect was seen at both the initiation and promotion stages of tumor development.

Such findings concur with those obtained from cancer cell cultures grown in the laboratory, in which curcumin blocked the growth of an impressive number of cells from human tumors, including leukemia cells, and colon, breast, and ovary cancer cells. These results seem linked to the blocking of certain processes necessary to the survival of cancer cells, which renders them incapable of resisting cell death by apoptosis. Other studies suggest that curcumin prevents the formation of new blood vessels by angiogenesis, thus depriving tumors of their source of energy.

Several studies have confirmed curcumin's cancer prevention potential by using experimental models where cancer is not induced by carcinogenic substances but by factors more representative of actual risks faced by humans. For example, in a model using a transgenic mouse that spontaneously developed polyps in the gastrointestinal tract, an important risk factor for colon cancer, the administration of curcumin was found to significantly slow down the spread of these polyps (by 40 percent). This effect would seem to be related in large part to the blocking of the dangerous progression stage of tumor development, which suggests that including turmeric in the diet of persons in whom these polyps are already present could help prevent the polyps from reaching a more advanced stage.

THE ANTI-INFLAMMATORY EFFECTS OF CURCUMIN

Colon cancer appears to be one of the cancers on which curcumin may have the greatest positive impact. This hypothesis is backed up by the observation that curcumin reduces levels of the cyclooxygenase-2 enzyme (COX-2), an enzyme responsible for the production of molecules that promote inflammation (aspirin and the now-notorious anti-inflammatory drugs Celebrex® and Vioxx® also inhibit this enzyme). It may well be that this property accounts for the beneficial effect that curcumin has on colon cancer. Studies carried out up until now indicate that these anti-inflammatories may reduce the incidence of this cancer. In fact, a recent study on the effect of administering curcumin orally showed a noticeable decrease in the number of inflammatory molecules formed by COX-2 found in the bloodstream of afflicted persons.

This effect is extremely interesting, especially in light of the latest results showing that synthetic anti-inflammatory drugs have potentially harmful side effects that may limit their future use in colon cancer prevention.

CURCUMIN AND PIPERINE: AN EXAMPLE OF CULINARY SYNERGY

Curcumin has at least one drawback: its low bioavailability (the extent to which it can be absorbed into the bloodstream). However, it is important to note that a molecule contained in pepper, piperine, increases the absorption of curcumin by a factor of 1,000, a property that can no doubt be exploited to maximize curcumin's potential health benefits (**see Figure 36, p.178**). Intriguingly, this is another case where common wisdom may again have anticipated scientific inquiry: pepper has always been an ingredient in curry powder. This example beautifully illustrates the concept of culinary synergy, or how eating a certain food may help to realize fully the potential health benefits of another eaten as part of the same meal.

▶ **Spices,** such as those shown here, do much more for us than flavor and color our food – they may also help to prevent chronic diseases such as cancer.

In summary

● **Turmeric and** its principal active ingredient, curcumin, possess numerous anticancer properties that may be responsible for the wide differences observed in the rates of many cancers in India and North America.

● **The relatively** low bioavailability of curcumin may be substantially increased by the presence of piperine (pepper).

● **The daily addition** of a teaspoon of turmeric to soups, salad dressings, or pasta dishes is a simple, rapid, and inexpensive way of providing a curcumin intake sufficient to help prevent the development of cancer.

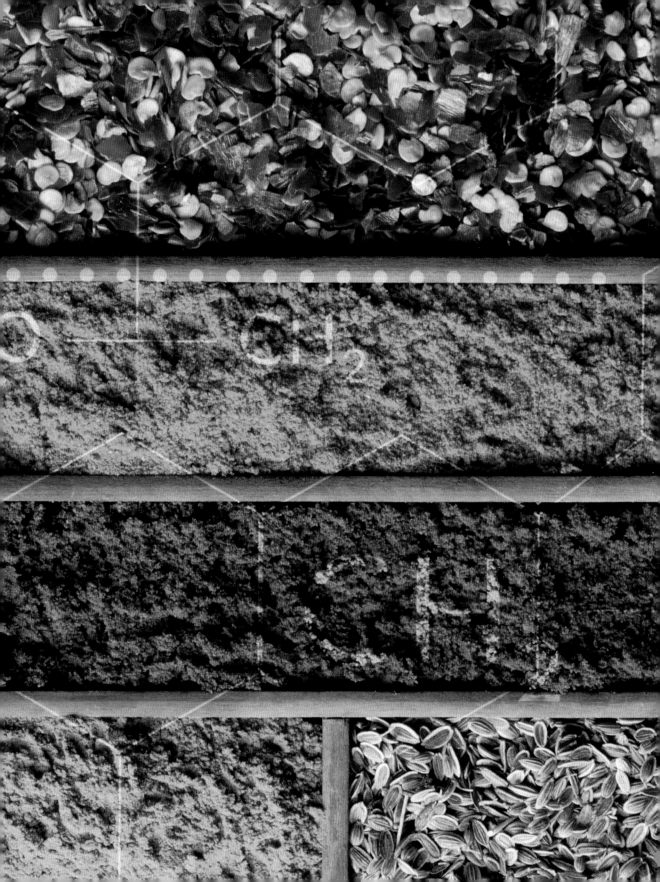

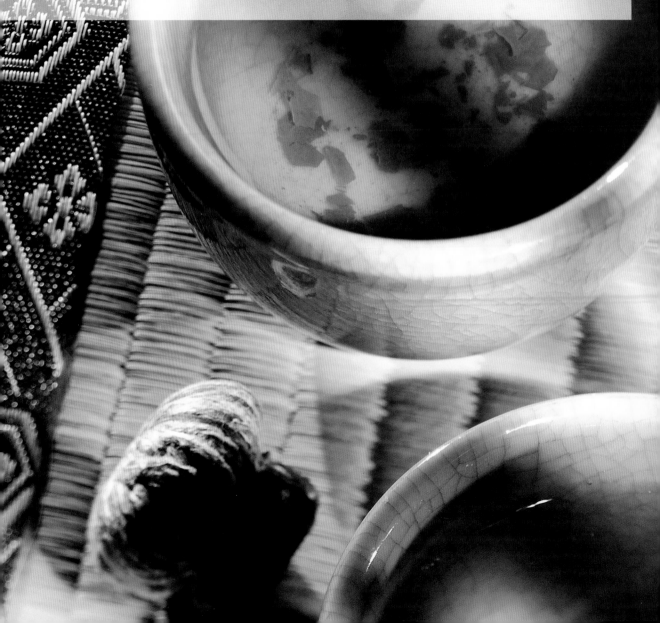

"Tea is an exquisite medicine that may prolong human life. The mountain country and the valleys where tea grows is holy and powerful."

Eisai, Kissa Yôjôki, *Drinking Tea for Health*, (1214)

Green Tea: Good for Soul and Body

When we in the West think of tea, it's probably black tea that comes to mind. It wasn't always this way – only in relatively recent times has black tea been preferred over green. The process of producing black tea from green strips the tea of its anticancer potential, so drink your tea green whenever you can.

It would be impossible to discuss adequately the concept of preventing cancer through diet without at some point giving the spotlight over to green tea. Much more than a simple hot beverage, green tea has become over the centuries a highly integral part of life and customs in Asian countries; from a gastronomic perspective, and as an element of hospitality and ritual, yes, but also as an essential substance in the prevention and treatment of disease.

Unfortunately, as is the case of other foods of Asian origin discussed in this book, green tea remains relatively little-known in the West; this difference, for some, explains the difference in cancer rates between Asians and Westerners. As we will see, green tea is an exceptional source of powerful anticancer molecules that make it a key feature of any diet designed to prevent the growth of cancer. And if that were not enough, it makes for a delicious, thirst-quenching remedy!

THE ORIGINS OF TEA

The discovery of tea was probably the result of many trials made by human beings to identify plants with specific healthful properties. According to Chinese legend, this discovery took place around 5000 BC, when the emperor Shen Nong, who had ordered water to be boiled to purify it, saw some leaves that had been floating on the wind fall into the hot water. The emperor was struck by the color of the water and the exquisite scent that it gave off, and decided to taste it. He was surprised to discover a drink rich in aroma that proved to have many other virtues.

Many historians consider the discovery of tea to have occurred only a few centuries before the time of Christ. The works of Confucius (551–479 BC), as well as other accounts written during the Han period (206 BC–220 AD), mention tea several times, although its use was restricted to medical treatments. It was only later that tea insinuated itself into daily life and became a custom, particularly during the Tang Dynasty (618–907 AD), when it was drunk both for pleasure and its regenerative properties, and when the art of growing and brewing tea became a noble pursuit, in the order of calligraphy, painting, or poetry.

The drinking of tea became so important by the end of the 8th century AD that the plant itself was subjected to a tax: the Chinese thus instituted a practice that was taken up much later by the British and was to have serious repercussions on the stability of that empire. (Hoping to increase revenue, the British made the error of applying an outrageous tax to certain foodstuffs, including tea, that were sold to their colonies. This practice provoked the anger of the American colonists, who retaliated in 1773 by dumping 342 cases of tea into Boston Harbor. The events of the Boston Tea Party, of course, led eventually to the independence of the United States from Britain.)

Japan, where the best green teas are harvested, also made important contributions to the flourishing fortunes of tea. Although the cultivation of tea was introduced there as early as the 8th century AD, it was not until the 12th century that it began to acquire the importance it now holds for the Japanese. The importance of tea in this culture is well illustrated by the *chanoyu*, or tea ceremony, a formal, very elaborate ritual based on the values of harmony, respect, purity, and tranquility. Although the ceremony is less frequently performed today, the spirit of *chanoyu* still informs the close

relationship that exists between green tea and the Japanese people.

GREEN AND BLACK TEA: WHAT IS THE DIFFERENCE?

Tea is made from the young shoots of the *Camellia sinensis* bush, a tropical plant that probably originated in India and was brought to China by way of the Silk Road. In the wild, plants may attain the size of trees, but they are cultivated as bushes for easy harvesting and to stimulate the growth of the young shoots and leaves. The three principal types of tea, green, black, and oolong, are all made from the leaves of *C. sinensis sinensis* (or *C. sinensis assamica*, in India), but their characteristics differ based on the process used to obtain the dried leaves (**see box, opposite**).

After water, of course, tea is the world's most popular beverage: 15,000 cups are drunk on the planet every second, which works out to 500 billion cups of tea every year, or an average of 100 cups per inhabitant. Today, black tea is favored over the others, accounting for 78 percent of world consumption, while green tea is preferred by only 20 percent of tea drinkers.

Black tea is primarily popular in the West, where it represents about 95 percent of tea consumed; however, in Asia these figures are reversed, with black tea consumpton lagging far behind that of green tea. Not all Asian countries show similar tea preferences; over 95 percent of the East's black tea is drunk in India, where it is a relatively recent phenomenon, one whose origins were strongly influenced by the colonial heritage left by the British.

In spite of their common origins, the chemical composition of green tea and black tea is completely different. In the course of the fermentation process used to make black tea, dramatic changes occur in the nature of the polyphenols that were originally present in the tea leaves: they oxidize to produce black pigments called theaflavins. This transformation has serious consequences; the oxidized polyphenols have very little or no anticancer activity. This is why green tea is by far the more important contender in the dietary cancer prevention race. If these differences are taken into account, it seems logical to assume that modifying tea-drinking habits could have a considerable impact on the number of cancers occurring in Western societies.

Is such a modification likely to happen? We think so, for the simple reason that green tea is already a part of our lives to some extent; the factors that led Westerners to prefer black tea over green were for the most part political and economic ones, and not related to any dislike we might have for green tea itself.

Indeed, when tea was first introduced into Europe in the 1600s, probably by Portuguese merchants, it was almost certainly green, since the fermentation techniques needed to make black tea, which the Chinese call *hong cha*, or

THE MAKING OF TEA

Green tea

Green teas undergo the least transformation of all teas; their processing is still done manually for the most part. Only three steps are required to make green teas, but each of these is crucial to the quality of the finished product. The first step is a brief steam roasting of the freshly gathered leaves, which allows for the deactivation of the enzymes that would cause fermentation in a few seconds, and for the conservation of the leaf's original color. After a cooling and drying period, the leaves are rolled to create tight little balls; the rolling breaks up the leaf cells and frees the distinctive aromas. The balls are then dried and dehydrated by rolling them into smaller and smaller balls, until they attain the shape of a needle. All of these steps, from the harvesting to the treatments the leaves are subjected to, determine the quality of the tea. For example, teas cultivated in direct sunlight, known as sencha, make for a more refreshing drink; those grown in shadow, or gyokuro, are milder. The first harvest of the year, in May, yields very fine, tender leaves that are used to make sencha and gyokuro. The summer harvest produces the leaves used to make bancha, a stronger-tasting tea which nevertheless contains less caffeine. Gyokuro teas are considered by connoisseurs to be among the finest green teas in the world.

Black tea

The processing of black tea resembles that of green tea, except that the roasting stage is carried out at the end of the process rather than at the beginning. The leaves are first blackened by exposing them to heat in order to reduce their water content and release the enzyme responsible for fermentation, polyphenol oxydase. They are then rolled to break the cell walls before fermentation, a reaction during which the polyphenols are converted to black pigments. The final step, roasting, halts the fermentation process by deactivating the enzyme and removing an excess of humidity. As is the case of green tea, the quality of the black tea obtained after processing is directly proportional to the skill of the tea-maker. One of the best-known black teas, Darjeeling, is also one of the rare black teas that still contains significant levels of catechins, the anticancer compounds associated with tea.

Oolong tea

This tea, less widely drunk than either green or black tea, is a "semi-fermented" tea. This means that its processing is similar to that of black tea, but with a shorter fermentation period. Oolong tea has properties that put it somewhere between green tea and black tea; the tea from Formosa (Taiwan), slightly darker in color than that of mainland China, is the most sought after.

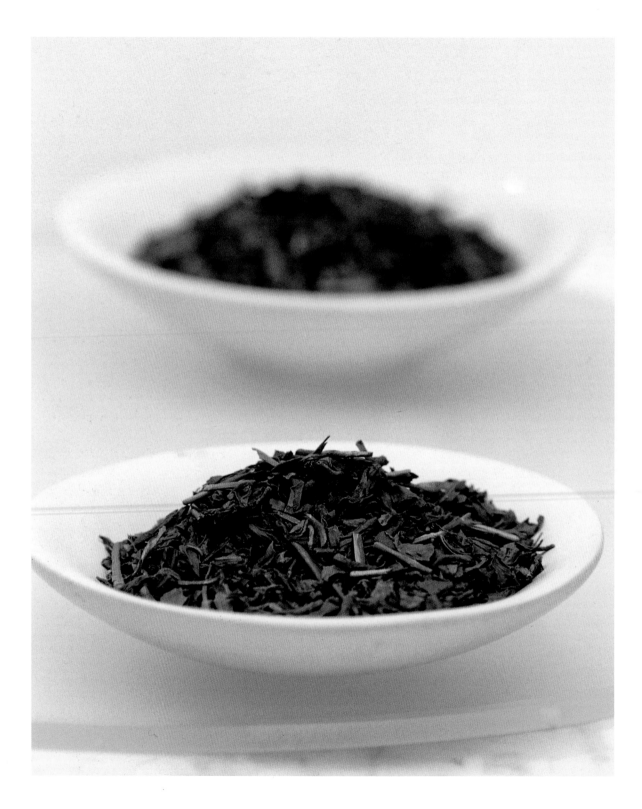

"red tea," had just made their appearance in China at the time of the Ming Dynasty (1368–1644) and were not yet widely known.

However, we could surmise that the long sea voyages towards those countries that imported tea might alter the delicate taste of green tea (the first delivery of tea to Canada, in 1716, took more than a year to arrive). The more robust black tea could more easily withstand transport over long distances without a noticeable change in taste; all the more reason for it to gain an early lead in popularity. Despite this problem and others, green tea was extremely sought-after in England well into the mid-19th century; it could also fetch a higher price because of its better appearance. This fact brought about some interesting marketing decisions: when the Chinese producers realized that green tea had the more pleasing shade, they tried to enhance the color of the leaves by adding different chemical compounds, probably copper salts, during processing. The ensuing scandal persuaded Britons to abandon green tea altogether; almost two hundred years later, green tea still accounts for only a small part of the British market. The colonization of India by the British led to the development of a large-scale local tea culture and established black tea as the European favorite. India today is the world's major supplier of black tea, with over 38 percent of total production.

Less single-minded than the British, North Americans drank as much green tea as they did black tea until the beginning of the 1930s, and even seemed to favor green tea slightly at one point. For example, Canadian archival documents from 1806 indicate that 90,000 pounds of green

◄ **Green tea** was once as popular in North America as black tea. Now that its anticancer potential has been discovered, green tea is becoming popular again.

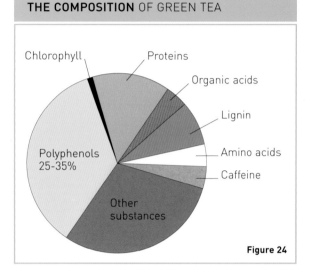

THE COMPOSITION OF GREEN TEA

Chlorophyll
Proteins
Organic acids
Lignin
Amino acids
Caffeine
Polyphenols 25-35%
Other substances

Figure 24

tea were imported into Canada that year, compared to only 1,500 pounds of black tea! It was only in 1931, at the start of the Sino-Japanese war for control of Manchuria, that green tea exports to North America fell off drastically and green tea-lovers were forced to switch to black.

Green tea, then, is not as foreign to Western culture as most people may have thought! We are convinced that it is possible to bring back this long-standing tradition so as to increase the consumption of green tea in North America and Europe. As we will soon find out, green tea is in a class by itself when it comes to anticancer activity. The simple act of replacing black tea by green tea could have a significant impact on the high cancer rates plaguing Western societies.

THE ANTICANCER PROPERTIES OF GREEN TEA

Tea is a complex beverage; it contains hundreds of chemical compounds that give it its distinctive aroma, taste, and astringency (**see Figure 24, above**). One class of compounds predominates, making up about one-third of the weight of the tea leaf: these are the polyphenols that are known as flavanols, more commonly known as catechins. Catechins are the heavyweights responsible for green tea's anticancer activity (see Figure 25, below).

Like all other polyphenols, catechins are complex molecules that play a very important role in plant physiology. They possess antifungal and antibacterial properties that allow the plant successfully to resist invasion by a large number of pathogens. Green tea happens to contain several catechins; the star among them, with the highest anticancer activity of all, is known as epigallocatechin gallate, or EGCG.

THE PRINCIPAL POLYPHENOLS PRESENT IN GREEN TEA

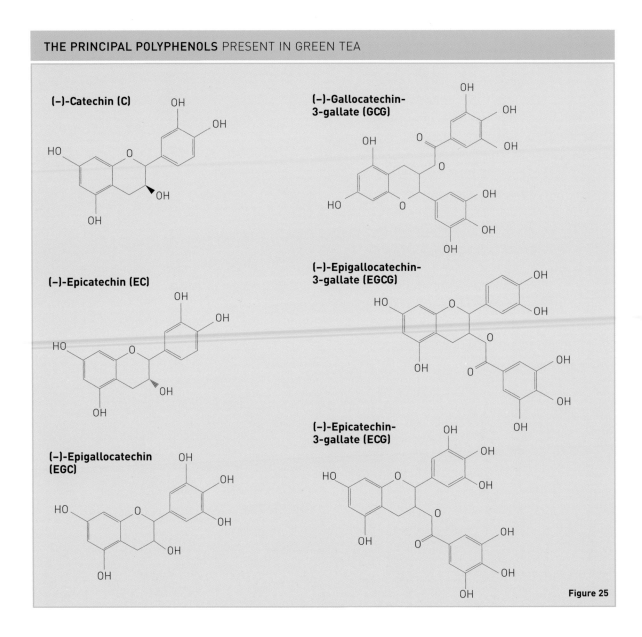

(–)-Catechin (C)

(–)-Gallocatechin-3-gallate (GCG)

(–)-Epicatechin (EC)

(–)-Epigallocatechin-3-gallate (EGCG)

(–)-Epigallocatechin (EGC)

(–)-Epicatechin-3-gallate (ECG)

Figure 25

It is important to note that the catechin content of green tea varies greatly depending on the area of cultivation, the diversity of plants used, the harvest season and, not least, the processing techniques that have been used. In other words, it is not necessarily because the label on a package says "green tea" that the product inside contains large amounts of anticancer compounds! When we analyzed different types of green tea, we observed important variations in the EGCG content released during the brewing period (see Figure 26, below). As a general rule, Japanese green teas contain far more EGCG than do Chinese teas.

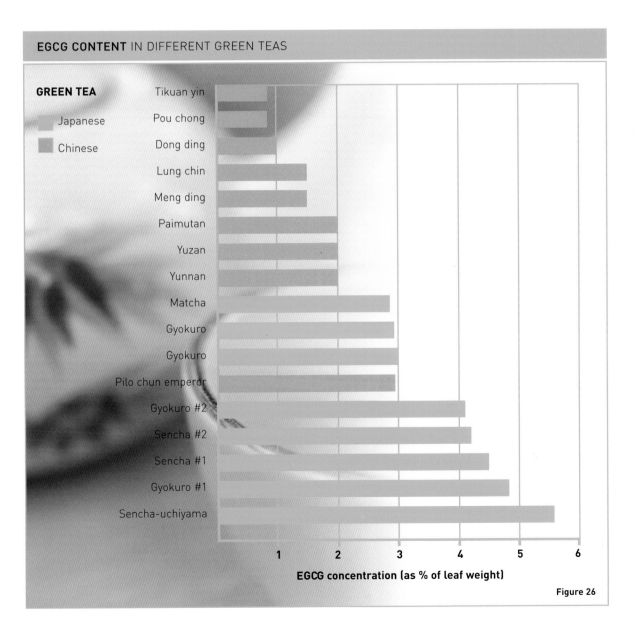

EGCG CONTENT IN DIFFERENT GREEN TEAS

GREEN TEA
Japanese
Chinese

Tikuan yin
Pou chong
Dong ding
Lung chin
Meng ding
Paimutan
Yuzan
Yunnan
Matcha
Gyokuro
Gyokuro
Pilo chun emperor
Gyokuro #2
Sencha #2
Sencha #1
Gyokuro #1
Sencha-uchiyama

EGCG concentration (as % of leaf weight)

Figure 26

THE **POLYPHENOL** CONTENT OF GREEN TEAS	
	mg polyphenols per cup
A cup of Ti Kuon Yin tea brewed for 2 minutes	9
A cup of gyokuro tea brewed for 10 minutes	540

Figure 27

Why brewing time matters

The brewing period (the time before drinking that tea leaves are steeped in boiling water) is also an important factor in final polyphenol content. An infusion time of less than five minutes allows the extraction of only 20 percent of the catechins that would normally be extracted after an infusion of 8–10 minutes. A tea of mediocre quality, brewed for less than five minutes, would therefore have a polyphenol content up to 60 times smaller than that of a fine-quality tea brewed for a sufficient period of time (**see Figure 27, above**). It goes without saying that these huge variations may have a significant impact on the potential anticancer effect associated with drinking green tea.

The very large variations in the composition of different green teas complicate any analysis that might be made of their chemopreventive effect in clinical studies. Nonetheless, studies carried out on green tea in recent years suggest beneficial activity in the prevention of cancer. The effect noted seems more pronounced in the case of bladder and prostate cancers. A slight protective effect against breast and stomach cancers was also observed, but these cases are more uncertain, as conflicting results were obtained in different studies. The differences are probably related in large part to extreme variations in the polyphenol content of green teas, and new studies seeking to clearly establish green tea's anticancer potential will have to take into account the amounts of polyphenols ingested rather than the volume of tea consumed.

In the meantime, there are many good reasons to believe that drinking green tea can significantly lower the risk of developing cancer. EGCG has been found to inhibit the growth of cancerous cell lines in vitro, among them lines from erythrocytic leukemia in mice, human leukemia, renal cancers, skin cancers, breast cancers, mouth cancers, and prostate cancers. These effects are significant because studies conducted on animals have shown that green tea prevents the development of many tumors triggered by carcinogens, mainly skin cancers, breast cancers, lung cancers, esophageal cancers, and colorectal cancers. However, the preventive effect does not seem to be restricted to cancers induced by carcinogenic substances, since the addition of green tea to the diet of transgenic mice who spontaneously develop prostate cancer considerably lowers the incidence of these tumors. The doses fed to the mice are comparable to those that humans would ingest by regularly drinking green tea.

GREEN TEA AND ANGIOGENESIS

One of the possible modes of activity of green tea that may most contribute to reducing tumor development is its extremely powerful effect on the process of angiogenesis. Of all the molecules naturally occurring in foods that have been identified up until now, our studies show that EGCG is the most powerful in blocking VEGF receptor activity, a key feature in the initiation of angiogenesis. Interestingly, the receptor inhibition occurs very rapidly and only requires quite small concentrations of the molecule: these small concentrations are easily reached by drinking several cups of green tea daily. The inhibition of angiogenesis almost certainly represents one of the principal mechanisms by which green tea may aid in preventing cancer.

History cannot be changed, but knowing the range of the anticancer properties attributed to green tea, one can only speculate that cancer might have become a far less serious burden in our society if our ancestors had continued to drink green tea instead of replacing it with black tea. The situation, though, is hardly irreversible. Those tea-lovers curious to explore new possibilities will be pleasantly surprised by the appearance of green tea, its thirst-quenching ability, and its weak caffeine content (four times less caffeine than black tea). Green tea represents far more than a single ingredient in a balanced diet designed to ward off disease: it can become the "soul" of such a diet, a symbol of the ease and pleasure of taking a daily dose of anticancer compounds in a calm, simple, and natural manner. The tea master Sen-no-Rikyu (1522–1591) said that the ritual of tea consisted of nothing more than the act of boiling water, making tea, and drinking it. With all that we have learned since then, we can add a fourth action to the master's list: preventing cancer.

In summary

- **Unlike black tea**, green tea contains large amounts of catechins, which are compounds that boast many anticancer properties.

- **To maximize** the preventive effects afforded by tea, select Japanese green teas, which are richer in anticancer compounds, and allow for an 8- to 10-minute brewing period, which favors an adequate extraction of the catechin molecules. Always drink freshly brewed tea and try to space out your three daily cups equally.

"Your taste of raspberry and strawberry,
Oh flower-flesh!
Laughing at the fresh wind kissing you
Like a thief"

Arthur Rimbaud, *Nina's Replies* (1890)

A Passion for Berries

At last, a food that tastes good has been found to be good for you! Berries, those perennial favorites, contain large amounts of certain phytochemicals that help prevent cancer. Eat berries in season and use the frozen kind out of season – they make a healthy treat all year long.

Synonymous with lightness and freshness, the source of the most subtle of perfumes, the most intense colors, and the most refined and sophisticated of flavors, berries belong to a very small class of foods whose place in our diet is due more to the passion we feel for their aroma and delicacy than to any nutritional value they might happen to possess! If you enjoy eating berries, you may be surprised to learn that these delicious fruits are treasure houses of phytochemical compounds with anticancer potential. Finally, something that is so enjoyable to eat turns out to have excellent health benefits!

THE RASPBERRY

The raspberry, from the 16th-century "raspis berry" (possibly from *raspise*, "a sweet rose-colored wine", or the Old French *raspe*, also meaning "raspberry") has long been a sought-after fruit; even the gods of Olympus ate and appreciated this extraordinary tasting berry. Greek mythology tells us that the young Zeus was prone to terrible fits punctuated by furious cries. Looking to calm him, Ida, the nymph who acted as his nurse, went to pick a raspberry from among the bushes growing on the mountain side in Crete, where Zeus had been hidden to protect him from the murderous instincts of his father Cronos. As she plucked the berry, Ida grazed her breast on the briar and bled onto the then-white raspberries, forever staining them a brilliant red color. This legend traveled across time; at the beginning of the 1st century AD, Pliny the Elder opined that Mount Ida, the highest summit on Crete, was the only place in the world where raspberries grew.

Although it is likely that the origins of the raspberry bush were in the mountainous regions of eastern Asia rather in Greece, botanists gave the berry the Latin name *Rubus idaeus*, or "Ida's briar," in honor of the old story.

As well as possessing undeniable qualities of taste, raspberries have long played a role in the medicinal traditions of different cultures: as an antidote to poison in Russia, or an anti-aging cure to the Chinese. Like the strawberry, the raspberry contains large amounts of a very powerful anticancer molecule, ellagic acid, and is therefore a very promising food from a therapeutic standpoint.

THE STRAWBERRY

The strawberry (from the Old English *streawberige*: *streaw*, "straw" and *berige*, "berry") bush is an extremely tough, resistant plant that grows wild in most regions of the globe, in North and South America as well as in Europe and Asia. Because of this widespread presence, it is likely that the origin of wild strawberry consumption is linked to the origins of humanity itself, a fact attested to by the presence of tiny strawberry seeds in prehistoric dwellings.

Named *fraga* by the Romans in honor of its exquisite scent (and from which we get the word "fragrance"), the wild or wood strawberry, *Fragaria vesca*, was picked only in underbrush; curiously, the Romans did not particularly appreciate the taste of the berry itself. As Virgil wrote in his Bucolics, "You, picking flowers and strawberries that grow so near the ground, fly hence, boys, get you gone! There's a cold adder lurking in the grass." It is likely that the pleasant rendez-vous made by young Roman adolescents while picking strawberries were probably of more interest to those concerned than the berries being picked!

The domestication of strawberries seems to have begun in France in the mid-14th century, as gardeners sought to transplant wild strawberry bushes into the royal gardens. The considerable efforts expended testify to a certain kingly passion for these berries: in 1368, Jean Dudoy, royal gardener to France's King Charles V, transplanted no fewer than 1,200 strawberry bushes into the royal gardens at the Louvre, in Paris. Indeed, the close relationship between strawberries and royalty is of long standing in French history. When King Louis XIII traveled to Aquitaine in 1622 to put down the region's Protestant rebellion, his daily meal consisted of strawberries in sweetened wine and a strawberry cream tart.

The strawberry we know today is very different from the one eaten in the time of French kings; it comes from selections that were made from two varieties of strawberry bushes foreign to Europe. At the beginning of the 1600s, French explorers returning from North America brought back an interesting variety, the Virginia, or scarlet, strawberry (*Fragaria virginiana*), which would be cultivated on a large scale in the hothouses of Versailles under both Louis XIII and Louis XIV, the latter enjoying the berries so much that he would eat them to the point of indigestion. Amédée-François Frézier, whose name may have predisposed him to play an important role in the history of the strawberry (the French word for strawberry is *fraise*), is the person most responsible for the existence of the strawberries eaten today around the world. An officer and cartographer in the Engineer Corps of the French Navy, Frézier was assigned in 1712 to put Spanish ports of call and fortified settlements on South America's Atlantic coast under surveillance. He noticed a type of strawberry bush that grew on the shoreline,

THE STRAWBERRY: MYTHS AND SYMBOLS

Although its origins in legend seem less poetic than those of the raspberry, there are many symbols, myths, and legends associated with the strawberry. For some Native American tribes, the souls of the dead would not forget the world of the living until they had found and eaten a huge strawberry that satisfied them and allowed them to rest in peace for all eternity. For Westerners, the strawberry's red color, tender flesh, and sweet juice, not to mention its resemblance to a heart, make it a synonym for love, sensuality, and temptation. The strawberry has also long been used as a beauty aid, for fighting wrinkles and toning the skin. The seductive Madame Tallien, an ambassador of Parisian fashion in the years following the French Revolution, regularly crushed twenty pounds of strawberries in the lukewarm water of her bath to preserve her skin's legendary freshness and firmness: an unthinkable waste of food that allowed her to display herself at the opera wearing only a sleeveless white silk tunic and no underwear!

Strawberries and allergic reactions

One of the only somber aspects of the strawberry is that this fruit, like chocolate, bananas, and tomatoes, stimulates histamine production by the immune system, often triggering false food allergies and causing a number of unpleasant side effects such as asthma or rashes. However, these pseudo-allergies do not involve the formation of specific antibodies and are not as dangerous as a real allergy to strawberries, which is quite rare (being fewer than 1 percent of all food allergies).

a bush bearing large, white berries later known as Chilean or beach strawberries (*Fragaria chiloensis*). Frézier managed to bring five plants back to France; although these bore no fruit, their flowers allowed botanists to cross-pollinate other species, particularly *F. virginiana*. This cross-pollination gave rise to the ancestor of the strawberry cultivated on every continent today, *Fragaria ananassa*.

The use of strawberries and of the strawberry plant in general for therapeutic purposes seems to be very old. The Ojibway of eastern Ontario prepared infusions of strawberry plant leaves as treatment for stomach troubles and gastrointestinal ailments such as diarrhea. Strawberries were exalted for more than their purgative properties: the famed Swedish botanist Carl Linnaeus was convinced that an intensive strawberry cure had miraculously healed his severe attack of gout. The French philosopher Bernard de Fontenelle, who died at the age of 100 (1657–1757), attributed the secret of his longevity to annual strawberry cures. If these anecdotes make us smile today, they do not contradict recent scientific results suggesting that strawberries may indeed be a food possessed of genuine therapeutic virtues, especially in regard to cancer prevention.

THE BLUEBERRY

A close relative of the European bilberry or whortleberry (*Vaccinium myrtillus*), the blueberry (*Vaccinium angustifolium*) is a species indigenous to northeastern North America; it did not find a place in the Western diet until the discovery of the New World by Europeans. Blueberries were food in ancient times. Native tribes revered the fruit, which they believed to be sent by the gods to save their families from famine. The newly arrived Europeans quickly adopted the blueberry as part of their diet and imitated Native American dietary customs, which included the blueberry in just about everything: soups, stews, and, of course, desserts.

American Indians used the blueberry as food but did not ignore its medicinal value. One particular remedy was a tea prepared from the plant's roots and used as a relaxant for pregnant women; another tea, made from blueberry leaves, acted as an overall tonic that also soothed colicky babies. The Ojibway and other Algonquin nations so believed in the calming power of the blueberry that they used the flowers to treat madness.

In Europe, the bilberry was used to cure common ailments such as diarrhea, dysentery, and scurvy. This berry has long been believed to treat circulatory problems successfully, as well as eye diseases such as diabetic retinopathy, glaucoma, and cataracts; some physicians still use it as a part of such treatments. This use becomes doubly interesting when we consider that diabetic retinopathies are caused by uncontrolled angiogenesis in the retina's blood vessels, an analogous phenomenon to that which supports tumor growth by triggering the formation of a new network of blood vessels (see Chapter 3, p.35). As we shall see later, recent scientific data suggests that a class of molecules known as anthocyanidins, which are found abundantly in blueberries and bilberries, could be responsible for the anti-angiogenic effects of these berries and thus help slow the growth of tumors.

THE CRANBERRY

Despite their rich red color and extremely acidic taste, cranberries belong to the Vaccinium family and are therefore close cousins of the blueberry and the bilberry. Like the blueberry, the cranberry has its own European cousin, *Vaccinium vitis idaea*, or lingonberry, but the best-known varieties are the North American ones: *Vaccinium oxycoccus* (small berries) and *Vaccinium*

macrocarpon (large berries), the latter being the variety that is now commercially cultivated.

The cranberry now occupies a relatively small place in the modern diet, except, of course, as an accompaniment to Thanksgiving or Christmas holiday turkey, a tradition stretching back to 1621, when the Pilgrims celebrated their first harvest in Massachusetts. However, Native Americans enjoyed cranberries in abundance; known as *atoca*, they were used in a wide variety of ways, primarily in the form of dried fruit as well as part of the recipe for pemmican, a mixture of dried meat and fat that was eaten over the winter months.

Without formal scientific confirmation of the fact, it seems that Native Americans benefited from the cranberry's high benzoic acid content, using it as a natural preservative that increased the conservation time of other foods. Today, while increasingly popular eaten as dried fruit, cranberries are still mostly consumed in the form of juice, which is a pity: commercial cranberry juice drinks contain large quantities of sugar and far smaller amounts of the phytochemical molecules that are responsible for the cranberry's beneficial properties.

Popular tradition ascribes a special, well-known role to cranberries in the treatment of urinary infection. Seeing Native Americans use cranberries to treat bladder and kidney disorders allowed early settlers to discover the therapeutic effects of these small berries. Remarkably, this piece of traditional medicine was again found to have a basis in science; American physicians later observed that certain compounds present in cranberries prevent the adherence of bacteria to the cells of the urinary tract, thus reducing the risk of infection in this tissue. Molecules found in both the cranberry and the blueberry may also play a role in cancer prevention.

THE ANTICANCER POTENTIAL OF BERRIES

Given that berries occupy a relatively small part of our diet, mostly due to their being a seasonal food, it is extremely difficult to determine precisely their impact on tumor development. In fact, there has been to our knowledge no important study on the possible relationship between the consumption of berries and the risk of developing cancer. Yet researchers interested in the anticancer activity of different foods often mention berries as potentially important players in cancer prevention. Let's see why this is.

Ellagic acid

Of all the phytochemical compounds associated with berries, ellagic acid is the one most likely to interfere with the development of cancer. This molecule is a polyphenol with a unique structure, found principally in raspberries, strawberries, and certain nuts, such as hazelnuts and pecans (see Table 12, p.122). However, although raspberries seem at first glance to contain higher levels of ellagic acid than strawberries, the ellagic acid in raspberries is 90 percent present in the seeds, while that in strawberries is 95 percent present in the pulp of the fruit. It is therefore possible, and even likely, that the ellagic acid in strawberries is more easily assimilated than that in raspberries.

With respect to this, it is interesting to note that a new variety of strawberry recently developed in Canada, which is called the "Authentique Orléans," contains very high levels of ellagic acid as well as other phytochemical compounds, probably making it the world's first nutraceutical strawberry.

The anticancer potential of strawberries and raspberries, the principal dietary sources of ellagic acid, has been studied using laboratory-grown cancer cells as well as in laboratory animals that have been subjected to substances that cause tumors to form.

Both strawberry and raspberry extracts are able to counter the growth of tumor cells, these effects being directly related to the quantity of polyphenols contained in these berries and not to their antioxidant potential. In animals, studies showed that a diet containing a relatively high proportion of strawberries or raspberries (5 percent of total diet) led to a significant decrease in the number of esophageal tumors triggered by NMBA, a powerful carcinogen.

The mechanisms by which ellagic acid interferes with the development of cancer resemble at first glance those described for a number of other foods. The currently available data tends to bear out this observation, indicating that ellagic acid prevents the activation of carcinogenic substances into cellular toxins, which lose their ability to react with DNA and induce mutations capable of triggering cancer. Ellagic acid may also increase cells' capacity to defend themselves against toxic aggression by stimulating their carcinogen elimination mechanisms. However, our own results indicate that ellagic acid could be an even more versatile anticancer molecule than expected. We have discovered that this molecule is an extremely powerful inhibitor of VEGF and PDGF, two proteins essential to the spread of tumor vascularization, the angiogenesis process described in Chapter 3. In fact, just as we observed for certain compounds present in

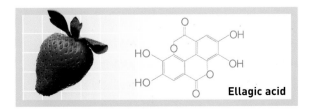

Ellagic acid

green tea, ellagic acid is almost as powerful as certain molecules developed by the pharmaceutical industry in interfering with the cellular phenomena leading to the formation of new blood vessel networks in tumors. Given the importance of angiogenesis in the development and progression of tumors, the anti-angiogenic activity of ellagic acid can only contribute to its anticancer potential; because of this, strawberries and raspberries are both worthy of special consideration in any strategy of cancer prevention through diet.

Anthocyanidins

Anthocyanidins are a class of polyphenols responsible for almost all of the vivid colors – red, pink, mauve, orange, and blue – found in many fruits and vegetables. These pigments are particularly abundant in berries, and especially in raspberries and blueberries, which can contain up to 500 milligrams per 100 grams of fruit. Daily anthocyanidin intake may attain 200 milligrams in enthusiastic berry eaters, making these compounds one of the most frequently ingested classes of polyphenols.

High anthocyanidin content, which includes proanthocyanidins (**see Table 14, p.124**), may be responsible for the very strong antioxidant potential found in berries. As seen in **Table 13, opposite**, of all the fruits analyzed, blueberries are in first place, closely followed by raspberries, strawberries, and cranberries, and far ahead of most of the fruits and vegetables that form a regular part of our daily diet.

We have already mentioned that it is not always clearly established to what extent the antioxidant properties of foods play a role in the development of cancer. In fact, some data exists to suggest that not only are anthocyanidins powerful antioxidants, they may also have another kind of impact on the development

Fruits	Ellagic acid (mg per serving*)
Raspberries (and blackberries)	22
Nuts	20
Pecans	11
Strawberries	9
Cranberries	1.8
Different fruits (blueberries, citrus fruit, peaches, apples, pears, cherries...)	Less than 1.0

ELLAGIC ACID CONTENT OF DIFFERENT FRUITS AND NUTS

* 1 cup (150 g) serving for fruits and 1 oz (30 g) for nuts, as suggested by the USDA National Nutrient Database for Standard Reference (www.nal.usda.gov/fnic/foodcomp)   **Table 12**

of cancer. For example, the addition of different anthocyanidins to isolated cancer cells cultivated in the laboratoary causes phenomena such as the cessation of DNA synthesis and thus of cell growth, leading to cell death by apoptosis. One of the anticancer effects of anthocyanidins may also be related to angiogenesis inhibition. We have discovered that delphinidin, an anthocyanidin present in blueberries, has the capacity to inhibit the activity of the VEGF receptor associated with angiogenesis, at concentrations close to those occurring in food. It is interesting to observe that this activity is

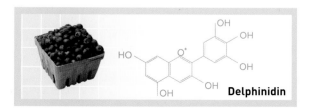

Delphinidin

probably not related to the antioxidant potential of delphinidin: malvidin, a very similar compound also found in large quantities in blueberries, possesses antioxidant activity equal to that of delphinidin, but displays no ability to interfere with the receptor.

Proanthocyanidins

Proanthocyanidins are complex polyphenols, created by many units of the same molecule, catechin, joining together to form a chain, or polymer, of varying length. These polymers are able to form complexes with proteins, especially proteins found in saliva, a property responsible for the astringency of foods containing these molecules. Although proanthocyanidins are found in abundance in the seeds, flowers, and skin of many crops, their presence in edible plants is somewhat limited (see Table 14, p.124). If we except cinnamon and cocoa, two extremely important sources of proanthocyanidins that cannot be consumed daily in large quantities (although some might take issue with this in the case of cocoa!), cranberries and blueberries constitute the richest food sources of these molecules. The other berries

ANTIOXIDANT ACTIVITY OF SELECTED FRUITS AND VEGETABLES

Fruits	Antioxidant activity per serving*	Vegetables	Antioxidant activity per serving
Wild blueberry	13427	Red bean	13727
Cranberry	8983	Artichoke heart	7904
Blackberry	7701	Russet potato	4649
Raspberry	6058	Red cabbage	2359
Strawberry	5938	Asparagus	1480
Apple (Red Delicious)	5900	Onion	1281
Cherry	4873	Sweet potato	1195
Plum	4118	Radish	1107
Avocado	3344	Spinach	1056
Pear	3172	Eggplant	1039
Orange	2540	Broccoli	982
Red grapes	2016	Boston lettuce	620
Grapefruit	1904	Sweet red pepper	576
Peach	1826	Frozen peas	480
Mango	1653	Canned corn	434
Apricot	1408	Sweet green pepper	418
Tangerine	1361	Tomato	415
Pineapple	1229	Celery	344
Banana	1037	Cauliflower	324
Nectarine	1019	Carrot	171
Kiwi fruit	698	Iceberg lettuce	144
Cantaloupe	499	Cucumber	60
Honeydew melon	410		
Watermelon	216		

* Expressed as "antioxidant power units", using a vitamin E-analog as a reference. The higher the value, the greater the ability of the food to act as an antioxidant.
Source: J. Agric. Food Chem. (2004), 52, 4026-4037.   **Table 13**

PROANTHOCYANIDIN CONTENT OF SELECTED FOODS	
Food	**Proanthocyanidin content** (mg per 100 g)
Cinnamon	8108
Cocoa powder	1373
Red beans	563
Hazelnuts	501
Cranberries	418
Wild blueberry	329
Strawberry	145
Apple (Red Delicious, with peel)	128
Grapes	81
Red wine	62
Raspberries	30
Cranberry juice	13
Grapeseed oil	0

Source: USDA Database for the Proanthocyanidin
Content of Selected Foods   **Table 14**

Cartier wrote in his journal of 1535: "The mouth becomes so putrefied, rotted through to the gums, that all the flesh falls off, up to the roots of the teeth, almost all of which fall out." Help arrived from a knowledgeable source: Domagaya, an Iroquois who had accompanied Cartier back to France after his first voyage, revealed the secret of a special tea prepared from the bark and needles of a conifer that was probably *Thuya occidentalis*, the Canadian white cedar. Upon drinking the tea, Cartier's shipmates were all rapidly cured; we now know that the miracle cure worked because of the presence of proanthocyanidins, which made up for the absence of vitamin C.

Proanthocyanidins (procyanidin C2)

As for cancer prevention: studies on the anticancer potential of proanthocyanidins are just beginning, but the results obtained so far are encouraging. In the laboratory, the addition of these molecules inhibits the growth of different cancerous cells, especially colon cancer cells, suggesting that proanthocyanidins may play a role in the prevention of this type of cancer. Similarly, it is being more and more clearly established that proanthocyanidins are able to disrupt the angiogenic development of new

discussed in this chapter contain much less, although the proanthocyanidin content of strawberries may be favorably compared to that of other foods rich in these compounds. It is also important to note that cranberry juice has a much lower proanthocyanidin content than does the whole fruit and cannot be considered a significant source of these molecules.

The proanthocyanidins are known primarily for their exceptional antioxidant power. This quality is discernible in the story of the French explorer Jacques Cartier's second voyage to America, during which his crew, forced to winter in what is now Quebec, was stricken with scurvy.

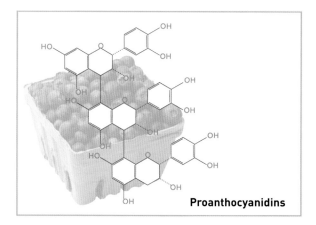

Proanthocyanidins

blood vessels and may therefore help keep microtumors in a latent state by preventing them from acquiring the blood vessel support network they need to grow. Finally, other studies have indicated that certain proanthocyanidins reduce estrogen synthesis and can thus help counter the harmful effects of elevated levels of these hormones. Even though the mechanisms responsible for these biological effects remain poorly understood, there is no doubt that proanthocyanidins possess extremely interesting characteristics from the cancer prevention perspective. Including foods that are rich in these molecules, such as cranberries, in the diet can only be beneficial.

Whether we consider their strong antiangiogenic activity or their antioxidant power, berries represent an important source of anticancer phytochemical compounds and deserve as such a special place in a diet oriented toward cancer prevention. Not to mention that including these delicious fruits in your family's daily meals should prove to be a popular decision!

In summary

- **Most berries** are an exceptionally abundant source of several classes of polyphenols that possess anticancer potential: ellagic acid, anthocyanidins, and proanthocyanidins.

- **Eating cranberries** should be preferred over drinking cranberry juice. Cranberries may be added to breakfast cereals or dried fruit mixtures.

- **Blueberries** and other berries may be eaten year round. Defrost frozen berries and use them as toppings for cereal or desserts.

"Too much of something is also a lack of something."

Arab proverb

Omega-3s: the Beneficial Fats

For years people have been conditioned to think of fats in the diet as bad, but some types of fat are actually vital for our health. The most important of these "good" fats are the omega-3 fatty acids. They are an essential ingredient in an anticancer diet, and they protect against heart disease too.

Over the last few decades, not too many people have had much good to say about fats. Although this negative reputation is well deserved in the case of animal fats, it is also true that there are certain fats of high quality that have very specific roles to play in normal body function (see **Figure 28, p.128**). In other words, we should not get hung up on the quantity of fats present in diet, but we should look instead at the quality of these fats. This is an important concept. Despite the large place occupied by fats in the Western diet, our largest nutritional deficiency, paradoxically, concerns the omega-3 fatty acids.

THE ESSENTIAL FATTY ACIDS

Some polyunsaturated fatty acids (omega-3s and omega-6s) are termed "essential" because our bodies are incapable of making them on their own; they must be supplied by our diet. For the omega-6 fatty acids, this requirement does not pose a problem, since these fats are present in large amounts in the major components of the modern Western diet – meat, eggs, vegetables, and various vegetable oils – and thus provide the body with sufficient linoleic acid (LA), the most important fat in this category.

However, an adequate supply of omega-3 fatty acids seems to be much more difficult to obtain from our Western diet. While the ratio of omega-6 to omega-3 fatty acids obtained through diet by the first human beings was probably around one to one, the ratio has now become more like twenty to one! This imbalance tipped in favor of omega-6 fatty acids may have negative repercussions on the development of some chronic diseases, such as cardiovascular

THE FATS IN FOOD

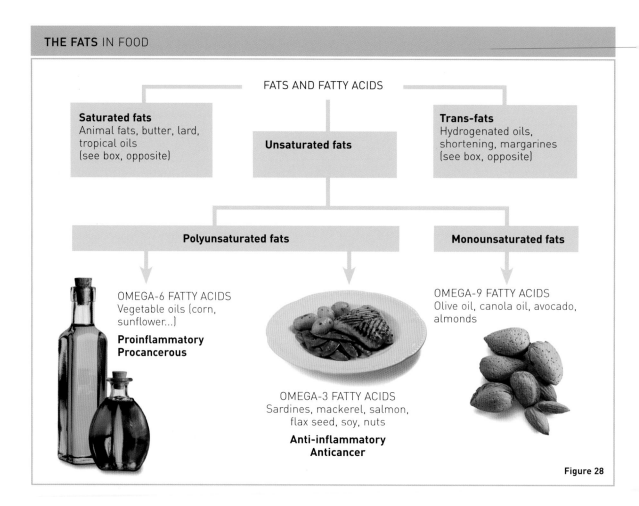

FATS AND FATTY ACIDS

Saturated fats
Animal fats, butter, lard, tropical oils
(see box, opposite)

Unsaturated fats

Trans-fats
Hydrogenated oils, shortening, margarines
(see box, opposite)

Polyunsaturated fats

Monounsaturated fats

OMEGA-6 FATTY ACIDS
Vegetable oils (corn, sunflower...)
**Proinflammatory
Procancerous**

OMEGA-3 FATTY ACIDS
Sardines, mackerel, salmon, flax seed, soy, nuts
**Anti-inflammatory
Anticancer**

OMEGA-9 FATTY ACIDS
Olive oil, canola oil, avocado, almonds

Figure 28

disease and cancer. This is because omega-6s are used by the body to synthesize molecules that play a role in inflammation, but omega-3s are needed for the synthesis of anti-inflammatory molecules. Increasing the intake of omega-3s while decreasing that of omega-6s may significantly reduce the risk of all inflammatory ailments, including cardiovascular disease and cancer.

OMEGA-3S: DHA AND EPA
A first hint indicating potential benefits of a diet rich in omega-3 fatty acids came from studies carried out on Greenland's Inuit population. Despite eating a diet based exclusively on the consumption of very fatty foods (such as seal blubber and whale meat) and lacking in fruits and vegetables, the traditional-living Inuit are spared from cardiovascular diseases for the most part. This protection is not genetic in origin (as Inuit emigrate, they become susceptible to these diseases), but seems to be related instead to the exceptional omega-3 fatty acid content of the seafood in the Inuit diet.

Fatty fish, in fact, such as mackerel, sardines, and salmon, are important sources of two omega-3 fatty acids, eicosapentanoic acid (EPA) and docosahexanoic acid (DHA). These fish synthesize the two fatty acids from alpha-linolenic acid (LNA), an omega–3 of plant origin that is present in large quantities in the phytoplankton they eat. LNA, which is not be confused with LA (the omega–6 that is ubiquitous in our diet), is found in certain foods, such as flax seeds, soy, and nuts (see Table 15, p.130). Researchers suspect that EPA and DHA synthesis from LNA does not take place very efficiently in

WHAT ARE THE TYPES OF FAT?

We have to admit that lipid, or fat, terminology is somewhat confusing. Here are some definitions that should help you better visualize what terms such as saturated fats, unsaturated fats, trans-fats, and omega-3 fatty acids refer to.

Fatty acids
Fatty acids can be compared to chains of varying length whose rigidity fluctuates according to different parameters.

Saturated fats
Saturated fats have straight, flexible chains; the molecules can pack together very closely. This means that saturated fats such as butter and other animal fats have higher melting points (it takes more heat energy to separate the tightly packed molecules). They occur in solid form both at room temperature and in the refrigerator.

Polyunsaturated fats
The structure of polyunsaturated fatty acids is different. The chains contain bends and kinks that create points of rigidity, so the molecules cannot pack together as tightly. This feature is responsible for the liquid character of vegetable oils.

Monounsaturated fats
Monounsaturated fatty acids fall somewhere between the two extremes of saturated and polyunsaturated fats: they contain a single point of rigidity. This is why olive oil, a rich source of these lipids, is liquid at room temperature but solid in the refrigerator.

Trans-fats
The properties of fatty acids can be modified: if polyunsaturated fatty acids are hydrogenated through industrial processes, their points of rigidity are destroyed, the geometry of the fatty acid chains is straightened, and the fat becomes a solid at room temperature (its melting point goes up). Margarine is produced using such processes. Unfortunately, this process causes modifications in the structure of the molecule, making it a trans-fat, one of a group of fats that are unknown in nature and that cause damage to cells.

Omega fatty acids
The term "omega," heard more and more often in recent years, comes from the way scientists identify the site on the molecule where the first rigid point in the chain is located. These points are numbered from the end of the chain. So omega-3 and omega-6 polyunsaturated fatty acids are fats whose first rigid point is found at the 3 and 6 positions, respectively. For the same reason, monounsaturated fatty acids are often referred to as omega-9s; the only rigid point in their chain occurs at the 9 position.

Omega   Point of rigidity (double bond)

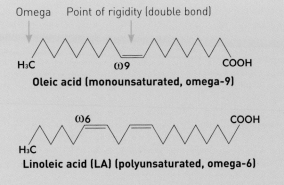

Oleic acid (monounsaturated, omega-9)

Linoleic acid (LA) (polyunsaturated, omega-6)

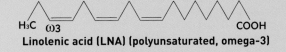

Linolenic acid (LNA) (polyunsaturated, omega-3)

the body when diet contains an excess of omega-6 fatty acids, as is now the case. This difficulty in synthesizing EPA and DHA arises because the enzyme factory that produces these acids from LNA is the same one that transforms LA, an omega-6, into inflammatory molecules. When diet supplies too much LA, the enzymes are submerged by an excess of lipids and fail to recognize and act upon the LNA that is present in far smaller quantities. Not only is the production of the omega-3 essential to cell equilibrium reduced, but there is excess

production of inflammatory molecules that can have harmful effects on body equilibrium.

One good way to reduce omega-6 fatty acid intake significantly is to use olive oil as the principal source of lipids (canola oil is also an option because of its better omega-6 to omega-3 ratio). If you wish to increase omega-3 content in your diet, it is enough to include as many plant sources as possible, such as flax seeds or soy, and to consume fatty fish (sardines, salmon, mackerel) regularly. These contain significant levels of pre-synthesized DHA and EPA that are ready for use by cells.

PRINCIPAL DIETARY SOURCES OF OMEGA-3 FATTY ACIDS

Plant sources	Linolenic acid (LNA) content (grams per serving)*
Fresh walnuts	2.6
Nuts	2.2
Walnut oil	1.4
Canola oil	1.3
Soybeans	0.44
Tofu	0.26
Animal sources	**EPA and DHA content** (grams per serving)*
Sardine	2.0
Herring	2.0
Mackerel	1.8
Atlantic salmon	1.6
Rainbow trout	1.0

*Servings of 1 tablespoon (15 ml) for oils, 1 oz (30 g) for nuts and 3½ oz (100 g) for tofu, beans, and fish. Adapted from USDA Nutrient Data Laboratory (http://www.nal.usda.gov/fnic/foodcomp) and from http://www.tufts.edu/med/nutrition

Table 15

BENEFICIAL EFFECTS OF OMEGA-3 FATTY ACIDS

The importance of increasing omega-3 fatty acids in the diet is linked to their beneficial effects on at least two ailments that afflict Western societies: cardiovascular diseases and cancer. A consensus has been arrived at concerning the benefits associated with the consumption of foods rich in omega-3s, particularly by people at high risk for developing cardiovascular diseases.

Studies show that omega-3s reduce the incidence of cardiac disease by lowering the risk of developing cardiac arrhythmia, the most common cause of sudden death from cardiovascular illness. These fats also reduce blood lipid levels, and the risks of the plaque formation characteristic of atherosclerosis are reduced accordingly.

However, the beneficial effects of omega-3s are not limited to cardiovascular diseases. More and more experimental findings suggest that these fatty acids may also play a role in cancer prevention. A certain number of studies that have examined a possible link between the consumption of fish rich in omega-3s and cancer have observed a decrease in the risk of developing breast, prostate, and colon cancers. The theory that omega-3 fatty acids may play such a role in the prevention of certain cancers is corroborated by other results obtained using animal models and isolated tumor cells.

Omega-3s versus omega-6s

Omega-6 fatty acids are known factors that may trigger the onset of cancer, but including omega-3s in the diet of laboratory rats causes the opposite effect. These compounds slow the development of breast, colon, prostate, and pancreatic cancers, while also increasing the effectiveness of chemotherapy medication.

The mechanisms involved in these protective effects may be related to two actions. The first is a decrease in the production of inflammatory molecules that disturb the immune system and favor the development of cancer. The second is a direct action on the cancerous cells by modifying their capacity to cheat death by apoptosis and preventing the development of the new blood vessels essential to their growth. So eating more omega-3-rich foods, such as fatty fish, can only have a positive impact on health, especially if this increased fish consumption is accompanied by a corresponding decrease in the consumption of saturated animal fats, such as red meats; it helps significantly reduce the risk of cancer. Changing your diet so as to increase omega-3 fatty acid consumption while reducing that of omega-6 fatty acids may certainly help to protect against cancer.

Easy ways to get your omega-3s

One tablespoon of freshly milled flax seeds added to breakfast cereal is an easy way of increasing omega-3 intake. Since fish are the best source of these fatty acids, eat two or three servings of fatty fish each week. They are also a good source of protein, vitamins, and minerals.

Unfortunately, some fish species do contain very small amounts of various toxic contaminants, but it should be stressed that in such tiny quantities, the benefits obtained by eating the fish are much, much more important than any harm that might be caused.

If this issue disturbs you, avoid eating large predatory fish, such as shark, swordfish, and tuna, more than once a week. Fish that are good sources of omega-3 fatty acids (salmon, sardines, and mackerel) contain only trace amounts of toxins. Choose wild salmon over farmed, because the latter are generally fed grains rich in omega-6 fats instead of algae and thus contain fewer omega-3 fats.

In summary

- **The greatest** nutritional deficiency currently affecting North American and European countries is the low intake of polyunsaturated fatty acids of the omega-3 variety.

- **Omega-3 fatty acids** are naturally extremely unstable, and it is preferable to use whole foods as a source of these lipids instead of omega-3 supplements.

- **Eating fatty fish** once or twice a week is one simple way of increasing omega-3 levels in the diet. Another is using a spoonful of freshly milled flax seeds as a topping for breakfast cereal.

"A world devoid of tomato soup, tomato sauce, tomato ketchup and tomato paste is hard to visualize... How did the Italians eat spaghetti before the advent of the tomato?"

Elizabeth David, *An Omelette and a Glass of Wine* (1984)

Tomatoes: the Prostate's Friend

The humble tomato is proving to be another important food in the anticancer kitchen. Tomatoes have so much going for them – they're not expensive, they're readily available, and their anticancer properties are enhanced by cooking. It's hard to believe they were once thought poisonous!

The tomato hails originally from South America, probably Peru, where it still exists in the wild. Yellow in color, and about the size of cherry tomatoes, Peruvian tomatoes were not eaten by the Incas. It was the Aztecs of Central America who began to cultivate the food they called *tomatl*, or "fleshy fruit," which they were already combining with sweet peppers to prepare what was doubtless the ancestor of salsa.

Discovered by the Spaniards who conquered Mexico in the early 16th century, the tomato was brought back to Spain, from where it made its way to Italy. Italians noticed the resemblance of this new *pomo d'oro* to the belladonna plant and the legendary mandrake, two plants with very powerful psychotropic effects, and this is why the tomato quickly gained a reputation as a toxic food. It was adopted instead exclusively for use as an ornamental climbing plant in Northern Europe. It "served commonly to cover outhouses and arbors, climbing gaily over top, clinging firmly to all supports.. Their fruit is not good to eat: they are useful only as medicine and pleasant to the touch or to the scent" (Olivier de Serres, the 17th-century French father of agriculture, agronomist to King Henri IV, in *Le Théâtre d'agriculture et le Ménage des champs*, 1600).

It was more than one hundred years later, in 1692, that the tomato made its appearance in an Italian cookbook; another century passed before its use in cuisine began to spread over the rest of Europe. The inhabitants of the New World showed the same reluctance to include the tomato in their daily diet, despite the example given by such famous tomato enthusiasts as Thomas Jefferson. The tomato as dietary staple

---

THE TOMATO: FRUIT, VEGETABLE... OR POISON?

Ancient beliefs held that the tomato was a dangerous thing. Although this may amuse us, we have to credit our ancestors for their sense of observation: the tomato does in fact belong to the Solanaceae, or nightshade, family, some of whose members, such as tobacco, belladonna, mandrake root, and datura, or angel's trumpet, contain very powerful, harmful, or fatal alkaloids. (Other members of this family include many commonly cultivated plants: potatoes, sweet peppers, eggplant, and petunias, to name a few.) Tomato plants contain one of these substances, tomatine, an antibiotic, which is abundantly present in the roots and leaves, less so in the fruit, and nonexistent in the ripened fruit. (All parts of the plant with the exception of the fruit are toxic. The same is true for other nightshade family plants.) The ambivalence of human beings toward the tomato comes across in its botanical Latin name, *Lycopersicon esculentum*; literally, "edible wolf-peach." The name was inspired by a German legend, which tells that local witches used hallucinogenic plants such as belladonna and mandrake to create werewolves.

So is it a fruit or a vegetable?
Finally, we should note that the tomato may be considered both a fruit and a vegetable. From a botanist's perspective, it is a fruit (a berry!), since it is produced as the result of the fertilization of a flower. However, from a horticultural point of view, the tomato is a vegetable, much as squashes are, with respect to its cultivation and the ways in which it is used. This classification is above all an economic one: an early American entrepreneur wishing to be exempted from the duties applied to imported vegetables tried to convince people that the tomato was a fruit. His formal request was officially rejected in 1893 by the Supreme Court, which ruled the tomato to be a vegetable.

---

did not enter into common use until the mid-19th century; today, it is a primary source of vitamins and minerals in the Western diet.

LYCOPENE, THE FACTOR RESPONSIBLE FOR THE TOMATO'S ANTICANCER PROPERTIES

Lycopene belongs to the vast family of carotenoids, an extremely diverse class of phytochemical molecules that are responsible for the yellow, orange, and red colors of many of our fruits and vegetables.

Since the human body is incapable of synthesizing carotenoids, these molecules must be obtained from plant sources in the diet. Certain carotenoids, such as betacarotene and betacryptoxanthin, are precursors to vitamin A, a vitamin essential for growth, while other family members, such as lutein, zeaxanthin, and lycopene, do not exhibit any chemical activity related to vitamin A and thus have other roles to play in body chemistry.

For example, lutein and zeaxanthin efficiently absorb the blue light in the spectrum and may protect the eyes by reducing the risk of age-related macular degeneration and cataract formation. The role of lycopene remains little understood, but many recent observations suggest that of all the carotenoids, it is probably the one with the greatest potential impact on cancer prevention.

Lycopene is the pigment responsible for the tomato's red color, and the tomato, whether considered a fruit or a vegetable, is the best dietary source of lycopene. As a general rule, tomato-based products constitute about 85 percent of all lycopene intake, with certain other fruits supplying the remaining 15 percent (see Table 16, opposite). The lycopene content of our cultivated tomatoes is unfortunately much lower than that of the original wild-growing species. Our current tomato, *Lycopersicon pimpinellifolium*, has 50 micrograms of lycopene per gram, compared to 200-250 micrograms per gram in certain wild species of tomato. This difference is due to the limited number of species used in hybridization procedures, which also reduce plant gene variability. Scientists hope that the reintroduction of the genetic baggage carried by wild species will increase the lycopene content in cultivated tomatoes, in order to reach levels capable of interfering with the development of cancer.

Lycopene levels and cooking methods

Products made from cooked tomatoes are particularly rich in lycopene. The rupture of cell walls exposed to heat allows for a better extraction of the molecule, and causes changes in its structure that let it be more easily assimilated into the body. Fats also increase the availability of lycopene, so cooking tomatoes in olive oil is an excellent way to maximize the amount of lycopene that can be absorbed. Incidentally, despite what the Reagan administration proposed in 1981 in trying to justify a decision to cut spending in school lunch programs, ketchup is not a vegetable! Its high lycopene content should not blind us to the fact that it is almost one-third sugar by weight.

LYCOPENE AND LOW PROSTATE CANCER LEVELS: WHAT IS THE LINK?

Countries with heavy tomato consumption, such as Italy, Spain, and Mexico, have much lower prostate cancer rates than do North America and the United Kingdom. Obviously, statistics such as these do not prove that the difference is due to tomatoes in the diet. For example, Asian cuisines do not as a rule include tomatoes, and

Asians do not as a group experience high prostate cancer rates. However, the data has inspired scientists to try to establish a link between a low incidence of prostate cancer and dietary intake of tomatoes. A certain number of studies have indeed suggested that individuals who consume large quantities of tomatoes and tomato-based products show a reduced risk of developing prostate cancer, especially the more aggressive forms of the disease. A word of caution: this tie has not been found in all studies conducted up until now; the great variability of lycopene content associated with different tomato products makes the demonstration of a beneficial relationship difficult. Conversely, studies focusing on large population samples and during which the risk of developing prostate

PRINCIPAL DIETARY SOURCES OF LYCOPENE	
Food	**Lycopene content** (mg per 100 g)
Tomato paste	29.3
Spaghetti sauce	17.5
Ketchup	17.0
Tomato sauce	15.9
Condensed tomato soup	10.9
Canned tomatoes	9.7
Tomato juice	9.3
Watermelon	4.8
Guava fruit	5.4
Raw tomato	3.0
Papaya	2.0
Pink grapefruit	1.5

Source: USDA Database for the Carotenoid Content of Selected Foods, 1998   **Table 16**

cancer was correlated with the consumption of lycopene-rich foods, such as tomato sauce, observed a decrease in risk of about 30 percent. The connection seems stronger for men aged 65 and over, indicating that lycopene may be better able to counteract the development of the prostate cancer associated with aging than the type that develops earlier, at around 50 years of age, which seems to be of genetic origin.

The mechanisms by which lycopene reduces the development of prostate cancer are not well understood. Like its close relative betacarotene, lycopene is an excellent antioxidant, but whether this property influences its anticancer effect remains unclear. According to the most recent findings, lycopene may hinder the development of prostate cancer by acting directly on certain enzymes that are responsible for the growth of this tissue. This action involves interfering with androgen signals (androgen is the hormone often involved in the excessive growth of prostate tissue) and disturbing the growth of cell tissue. Since the lycopene that is absorbed accumulates in the prostate area, the molecule seems to be ideally located to prevent an excess of cancer cell growth.

LYCOPENE AND CANCER IN GENERAL

Although most research on the anticancer effect of tomatoes has been concentrated on the prevention of prostate cancer, it seems likely that tomatoes might play a more general role in the prevention of other cancers. Since the molecular mechanisms responsible for the development of various cancers are often very similar, and it is reasonable to think that lycopene might also interfere with other cancers besides prostate cancer.

In summary, eating tomato-based products is an excellent way to reduce the risk of developing prostate cancer. Tomato sauce represents the ideal for this, since it contains high levels of lycopene in a form that that is easily absorbed. Eating two tomato sauce-based meals per week may lower your risk of developing prostate cancer by up to 25 percent. And don't forget the garlic!

▶ **Eating tomatoes** and tomato-based sauces regularly can be a delicious and inexpensive way to reduce the risk of prostate cancer, and possibly other cancers.

In summary

- Lycopene, a phytochemical, is the compound responsible for both the tomato's bright red color and its anticancer potential.

- Lycopene's anticancer activity is maximized by cooking tomatoes in the presence of vegetable fats, such as in sauces made with tomato paste and olive oil.

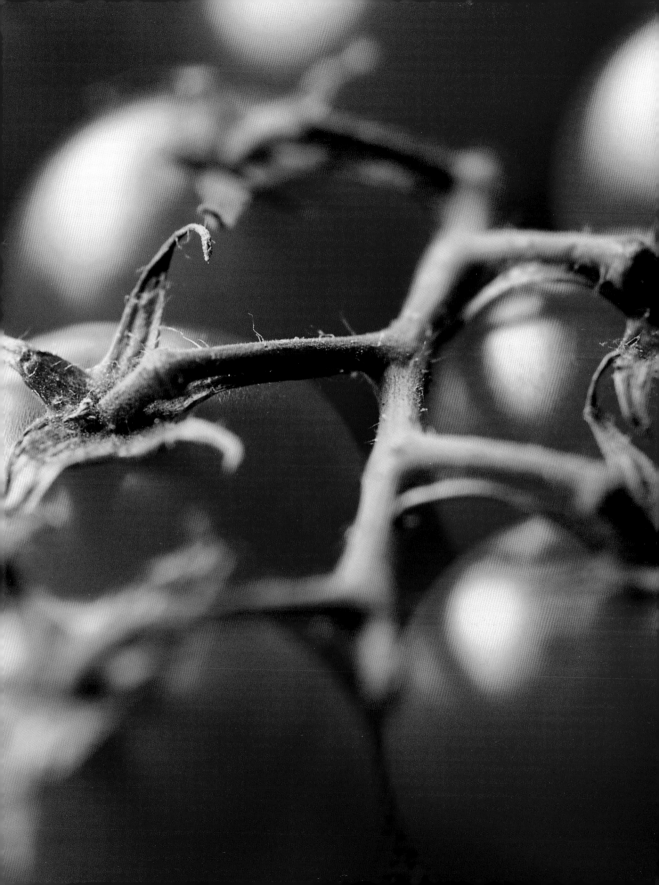

"So, when you hold the hemisphere
of a cut lemon above your plate,
you spill a universe of gold,
a yellow goblet of miracles…"

Pablo Neruda, "Ode to the Lemon," in *Elemental Odes* (1954)

Anticancer Fruits with Zest

Once a luxury food available only to the rich, citrus fruit is now a part of many people's daily diet. It has long been recognized that citrus fruit is high in vitamin C, but it has only recently been shown that it is also a valuable addition to a diet designed to help prevent cancer.

Citrus fruits, such as lemons, oranges, grapefruit, and mandarins (**see box, p.140**), belong to the sour-tasting, acidic Citrus genus in the orange family, Rutaceae. They are also known as *hesperidia* in reference to Hercules's eleventh labor, which had the Greek hero plucking three golden apples from a tree in a garden guarded by the Hesperides, the nymphs of the evening. The term "hesperidia" is in common use today only in the perfume industry, where it designates the essential oils obtained from citrus plants.

All citrus fruit originated in Asia, particularly in India and China, where they were cultivated at least 3,000 years ago. Europe had to wait for its explorers to find their way to the Asian continent and back to herald the arrival of the first citrus fruits in the West: the citron, or cedrat (*Citrus medica*), imported by Alexander the Great in the 4th century BC, or the sour or bitter orange (*Citrus aurantium*) introduced by the Arabs in the 1st century AD. Lemon trees were planted in 13th-century Spain and orange trees in 15th-century Portugal; mandarin trees were brought to Provence and North Africa in the 1800s. Long considered exotic fruit, citrus fruits now belong in the diet of the vast majority of countries and cuisines; a billion citrus trees producing close to 100 million metric tons of fruit every year are cultivated around the globe.

THE PHYTOCHEMICAL COMPOUNDS IN CITRUS FRUITS

Everyone, it seems, is now aware that citrus fruits are an abundant source of vitamin C. What is less well known is that citrus fruits also contain several phytochemical compounds that are in all likelihood responsible for their anticancer properties. For example, the orange contains almost 200 different compounds, among them about 60 polyphenols as well as several members of a very fragrant class of molecules, the terpenes.

Citrus fruits are the only plants containing significant amounts of a group of polyphenols known as flavanones, molecules responsible for the famous anti-scurvy effects that have long been associated with all citrus fruits.

One of these molecules, called hesperidin, was even known for a time as "vitamin P" because it acts to preserve capillary blood vessel integrity by strengthening and toning blood vessels and reducing their permeability. Since inflammatory processes in the body are characterized by an increase in blood vessel permeability, this indicates that these polyphenols are in fact also anti-inflammatory molecules, whose action could well contribute to preventing the development of cancer.

PRINCIPAL CITRUS FRUITS

The orange (*Citrus sinensis*)
Although the orange came to us originally from China, the word "orange" comes from the Arabic *narandj*, and further back, from the Sanskrit *nagarunga*, meaning "fruit beloved by elephants." Sweet oranges were introduced to the West in the 15th century by the Portuguese, who turned their cultivation into a local specialty and greatly contributed to their popularity. During his second voyage, Christopher Columbus brought orange seeds to the New World, beginning orange cultivation in the Americas. Back in France, the strawberry-loving King Louis XIV liked oranges just as much and had the famous "orangeries" at Versailles constructed to grow his private supply. Still considered a luxury at the beginning of the 20th century, the orange is the most commonly eaten citrus fruit in the world today, representing up to 70 percent of world citrus production.

The grapefruit (*Citrus paradisi Macfadyen*)
The grapefruit we know today is in fact a variety of pomelo created by the hybridization of the orange with an earlier variety of grapefruit. The "real" grapefruit (*Citrus grandis*) was known as *pomplemoes*, meaning "large lemon" in Dutch, a name they gave to the oversize pear-shaped fruit they had brought from Malaysia in the 1600s. So what is now sold under the name of pomelo is a grapefruit, while our "grapefruit" is really a pomelo!

The lemon (*Citrus limon*)
The lemon probably also originated in China and India, near the Himalayas, and was introduced into Europe by Arabs in the 12th century. Lemons should not be confused with citrons (*citron* means "lemon" in French!), another ancient fruit brought to the Mediterranean basin by Alexander the Great. According to such reliable authors as Theophrastus, Democritus, and Virgil, it was often used as an antidote to poison. As for the lemon, it was quickly discovered to be effective against scurvy, but it was not until the 15th century that it truly became part of the European diet. Despite its similar appearance and similar treatment by chefs, the lime (*Citrus aurantifolia*) is a different species, of Malaysian origin, that requires a more tropical climate than the lemon to flourish.

The mandarin (*Citrus reticula*)
The mandarin, whose name probably comes from the similarity of its color to that of the silk robes of Chinese courtiers, or mandarins, probably also hails from Southeast Asia. It was domesticated in China about 2,500 years ago. Cultivated on the shores of the Mediterranean from the beginning of the 19th century, the mandarin saw its popularity grow thanks to the development, in 1902, of its most famous hybrid, the clementine. Today, mandarins, tangerines, and clementines represent 10 percent of all citrus grown in the world.

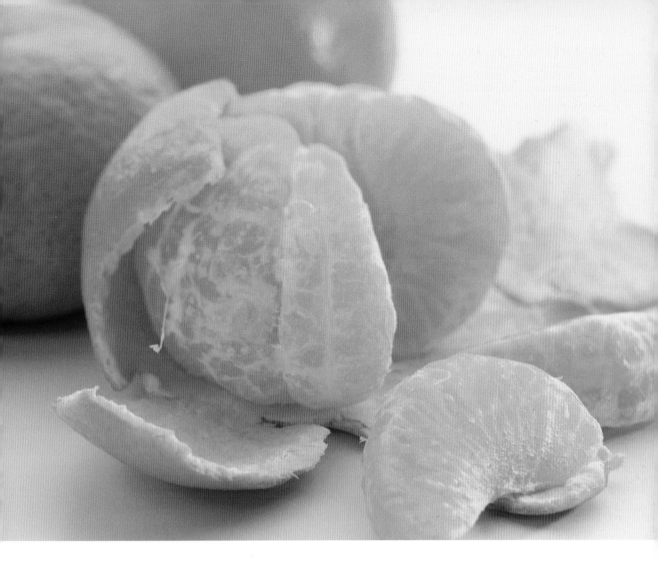

THE ANTICANCER PROPERTIES OF CITRUS FRUITS

Studies conducted in different parts of the world have succeeded in demonstrating a link between citrus consumption and a decrease in the risk of developing certain kinds of cancers. This relationship is particularly convincing in the case of digestive tract cancers, such as esophageal, mouth, larynx, and pharynx cancers, as well as stomach cancers, for which a decrease on the order of 40–50 percent was observed.

However, it is likely that other cancers can also be targeted by citrus. In recent findings, children who regularly consumed orange juice in the first two years of life had a reduced risk

▲ **Citrus fruits,** such as oranges, have abundant health benefits, and lately scientists have discovered that they can help protect against cancer too.

of later developing leukemia. These encouraging results have yet to be confirmed, but once again, they bear witness to the impact that diet can have on the development of certain kinds of cancers, from early childhood onward.

How does citrus fruit interfere with cancer?

In many respects, these observations agree with laboratory experiments in which the principal chemical compounds present in citrus, polyphenols and terpenes, have been identified many times as molecules that are able to interfere with processes leading to cancer. Even if the mechanisms involved in these events remain largely unclear, certain data suggests that phytochemical compounds in citrus fruit block tumor growth by direct action on the cancerous cells, restricting their ability to reproduce.

It is also very likely that one of the major anticancer effects of citrus is related to their modulation of the body's carcinogenic substance detoxification systems. The interaction of citrus fruits with these systems is nicely illustrated by the surprising effect that grapefruit juice can have on the metabolism of certain drugs.

In the course of a study intended to determine the impact of alcohol on the effectiveness of a commonly prescribed cardiac arrhythmia medication, researchers accidentally discovered that the grapefruit juice used to mask the taste of the alcohol was responsible for doubling the amount of medication absorbed into the bloodstream and thus increasing the number and severity of side effects. A similar effect was observed for statins, a class of medication used to lower blood cholesterol.

These observations show to what extent citrus fruit can regulate the systems involved in the metabolism of foreign substances in the body. We now know that these effects are due in large part to a molecule from the class of coumarins, deoxybergamottin, which blocks the liver enzyme responsible for drug metabolism (cytochrome P4503A4).

This particular behavior of molecules associated with citrus fruit is important. It may even turn out to be crucial to fulfilling the potential of the anticancer properties of other fruits and vegetables. All of the anticancer molecules of dietary origin described in this book are metabolized and eliminated from the body by the same enzymatic systems involved in drug metabolism. In other words, the inhibition of these systems by the phytochemical compounds in citrus fruit has the immediate effect of slowing down metabolism. The concentration of anticancer compounds in the bloodstream thus increases considerably, as does their potential activity.

THE MANY BENEFITS OF EATING CITRUS FRUITS

In summary, citrus fruits should not be seen solely as excellent sources of vitamin C, but also as foods capable of supplying the body with several anticancer phytochemical compounds. The many compounds present in these fruits act directly on cancerous cells, stopping their progression. They also exercise beneficial action as anti-inflammatories and by modifying the absorption and elimination of other substances. The daily consumption of citrus fruit, in the form of whole fruit or juice, is a simple and effective way of adding zest to a diet oriented toward cancer prevention.

In summary

- **Citrus fruits** are essential foods for cancer prevention. This is due to their capacity to act directly on cancerous cells as well as their potential for enhancing the anticancer effects of other phytochemical compounds present in diet.

- **Citrus fruit** consumption, whether in the form of whole fruit or juice, supplies the body with an incomparable source of specific anticancer molecules, while also providing the necessary daily requirements of many vitamins and minerals.

"A little wine is an antidote to death; in large amounts, it is the poison of life."

Persian proverb

In Vino Veritas

Surprisingly perhaps, red wine has been shown to be powerful ally in the fight to prevent some chronic illnesses, cancer among them. Although more research needs to be done, it seems clear that drinking red wine moderately as part of your daily diet can enhance health and longevity.

The grape is one of the most ancient and common fruits in the world. Fossil analysis indicates that wild vines existed more than 65 million years ago. Aided by the global warming of the time, they eventually spread over the entire surface of the globe some 25 million years ago, turning up in such unexpected places as Alaska and Greenland. This distribution became more limited over the course of subsequent glacial eras, so that ten thousand years ago, wild grapevines were for the most part concentrated in the Caspian Sea region corresponding to present-day Georgia and Armenia.

HOW WINE WAS DISCOVERED

Grapes are very sweet and thus subject to rapid fermentation, and it is likely that the proximity of humans and wild vines led to the discovery and preparation of the first beverages made by the fermentation of grapes. No one knows if the unique taste of these first "wines" was at the heart of efforts later made to domesticate the vines, but according to analysis of the seeds of the oldest cultivated grape known today, this domestication occurred some 7,000 to 5,000 years before Christ. It probably took place first in the Caucasus and then later further south, in Mesopotamia, where amphorae stained with wine dating from 3500 BC have been excavated.

This primitive viticulture was later considerably developed by the Egyptians, who considered wine a gift from Osiris, the god of resurrection. This status is reflected in the many frescoes decorating funeral chambers from the Third Dynasty onward (2686-2613 BC). Limited in its use to the Egyptian aristocracy, wine was produced in even greater quantities by the ancient Greeks, who spread its production and use around the Mediterranean basin. The whole of Greek society reserved a special place for wine, whose importance was symbolized by the cult of Dionysus, the Greek god of wine and intoxication. After the Roman conquest, Dionysus was replaced by Bacchus and the successors to the Greeks carried forward the culture and commerce of wine, not only in Italy, but on the Mediterranean coasts of France and Spain. More than two thousand years later, these regions remain the world's principal wine-producing areas.

THE BENEFICIAL EFFECTS OF WINE ON HEALTH

With the exception of tea, no beverage is as inextricably linked to human civilization as wine. If its exhilarating side has certainly made it an inescapable aspect of celebrations and festive rituals, it is interesting to note the extent to which wine has always been regarded as beneficial to health.

Wine, wrote Hippocrates, the founder of medicine, "... is a wonderful thing apt in health as well as in illness, if prescribed by necessity and in certain amounts in compliance with the individual build." He did not hesitate to recommend it in the treatment of many ailments. This therapeutic outlook on wine was shared by ancient Rome, where Pliny the Elder (23-79 AD), author of the voluminous *Natural History* (*Naturalis historia*) that we have already cited, also thought that "wine alone and of itself is a remedy; it nourishes the blood, pleases the stomach and calms worry and care."

The eruption of Mount Vesuvius in 79 AD prevented the unfortunate Pliny from going on about the virtues of wine, but these beliefs gained in importance and influence through the Middle Ages, as wine became an integral part of medical practice. The treatises of Europe's first medical school, founded in Salerno, near Naples, in the 10th century, mention that "pure wine has multiple benefits... and gives robust health in life... drink little of it, but let that be good." Such recommendations were still in vogue a few centuries later, at the University of Montpellier in France, which was then reputed to have the finest medical school in Europe. Circa 1221, fully half of the "medicinal recipes" listed in its learned works contained wine as an ingredient.

One might think that these ancient beliefs and customs, based more on intuition rather than on true medical science, would have disappeared over the centuries that followed. Far from receding, the place of wine in European medicine did not cease to expand until the 19th century. Even Louis Pasteur, already a celebrated microbiologist, considered wine to be "the healthiest and most hygienic beverage there is."

The scientific evidence

It was only at the end of the last century that concrete evidence of wine's potential health benefits was gathered. In the course of a study focusing on the factors responsible for mortality in cardiac disease patients, the French, in spite of a lifestyle and diet that boast many of the known risk factors for cardiovascular disease (high cholesterol levels, hypertension, smoking), were found to have an unusually low mortality rate from these diseases, much lower than other nationalities with roughly similar levels of the same risk factors. French people have a lipid (fat) intake similar to that of the Americans or the British, but they experience almost two times fewer heart attacks or other coronary events causing premature death. The major difference between the French and the Anglo-Saxon diets is the relatively high wine consumption of the French. This fact led to scientists positing the existence of the so-called "French paradox," the idea that consumption of wine, and particularly of red wine, might be related to lower mortality rates from cardiac disease.

RED WINE AND LOWER MORTALITY RATES

Numerous studies have pointed out that people who consume moderate amounts of alcohol on a daily basis have a mortality risk lower than either those who abstain from alcohol or those who drink to excess. The analysis of over fifty epidemiological studies conducted on the mortality rates of Western populations illustrates the existence of a response to alcohol that may be represented by a J-shaped curve (**see Figure 29, right**). Moderate quantities of alcohol (two to four glasses of about 120 ml each of wine per day for men and one or two glasses for women) significantly diminish the risk of death by 25–30 percent, for all causes of death. However, when these amounts are exceeded the mortality risk increases very rapidly.

Alcohol: a double-edged sword

The positive effect of moderate ethanol intake seems to be twofold: it causes an increase in HDL ("good" cholesterol) blood levels (a key factor in protection against cardiovascular disease), and it also decreases the tendency of blood to form clots by inhibiting blood platelet aggregation. Conversely, high doses of alcohol cause considerable damage to cells and substantially increase the risks of developing cancer. The graph represents this tendency by a sharp rise in mortality risk. Alcohol offers the perfect example of a double-edged sword that must be wielded intelligently if we are to benefit from its potentially healthful effects.

If alcohol at low doses is beneficial, this benefit seems much more pronounced for moderate wine drinkers. When mortality rates related to cardiovascular disease in eighteen countries were analyzed as a function of the amount of wine consumed by the inhabitants of these countries, it was observed that the mortality rate was much lower in countries with high wine consumption, such as France and Italy, and higher in countries such as England and the United States, where wine is not traditionally part of diet (**see Figure 30, p.148**).

A similar conclusion was reached in a recent synthesis of thirteen studies conducted on a total of 210,000 people. When the impact of red wine consumption on the risk of cardiovascular disease was evaluated in these subjects, it was

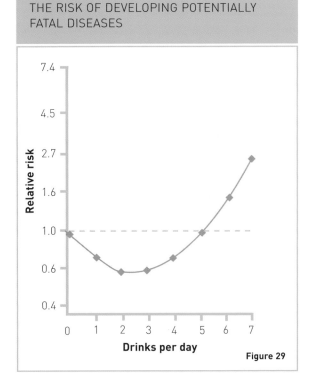

EFFECT OF ALCOHOL CONSUMPTION ON THE RISK OF DEVELOPING POTENTIALLY FATAL DISEASES

Relative risk

Drinks per day

Figure 29

apparent that moderate wine drinkers have about 30 percent fewer risks of being affected by these ailments.

Likewise, a Danish study showed that moderate wine consumption induced a 40 percent decrease in the risk of death related to cardiovascular disease, along with a 22 percent decrease in cancer mortality risk. These effects were much more pronounced than the effects that were observed for the moderate consumption of other types of alcoholic beverages, such as beer and spirits. It can be put very simply: moderate wine drinkers live longer than teetotalers, longer than heavy drinkers, and longer than drinkers who prefer other alcoholic beverages to wine.

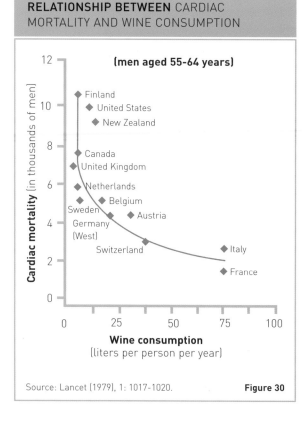

RELATIONSHIP BETWEEN CARDIAC MORTALITY AND WINE CONSUMPTION

(men aged 55-64 years)

Cardiac mortality (in thousands of men)

Wine consumption (liters per person per year)

Source: Lancet (1979), 1: 1017-1020. **Figure 30**

WHY IS RED WINE SO SPECIAL?

It may seem surprising that consumption of an alcoholic beverage leads to such a reduction in mortality rates from serious diseases, but it is important to understand that red wine is not an alcoholic beverage like any other. On the contrary – red wine is perhaps the most complex beverage in all of the human diet. This complexity is due to the long process of grape fermentation, which causes important changes in the chemical composition of the initial fruit pulp, allowing the extraction of certain molecules while modifying the structure of others.

The final yield is impressive: hundreds of distinct molecules, notably polyphenols, that are present in a bottle of red wine, one liter of which may contain up to 2 grams of polyphenols (**see Table 17, opposite**).

The importance of polyphenols in red wine

Polyphenols are found primarily in the skins and seeds of grapes. This means that much greater quantities of valuable compounds are extracted during the fermentation process leading to red wine, since, by definition, the skins and seeds are rapidly removed from the fermentation process when white wine is made.

Among the hundreds of polyphenols found in red wine, resveratrol is the one currently attracting the greatest interest as the molecule responsible for the health benefits associated with the moderate consumption of red wine. Although this molecule, quantitatively speaking, is a relatively minor component in wine (1 to 7 mg per liter compared to 200 mg per liter for proanthocyanidins, for example), resveratrol is found exclusively in red wine and may thus be seen as at least part of a plausible explanation for the benefits that red wine seems to confer on people's health.

THE PRINCIPAL PHYTOCHEMICAL COMPOUNDS IN WINE		
Phytochemical compounds	**Average concentration** (mg per liter)*	
	Red wine	**White wine**
Anthocyanidins	281	0
Proanthocyanidins	171	7.1
Flavonols	98	0
Phenolic acids	375	210
Resveratrol	3	0.3
Total	1200	217

*Given the extreme variability of the phytochemical composition of wines, the concentrations listed represent averages of currently available values.
Source: Annu. Rev. Nutr. (2000) 20: 561-593.

Table 17

This special interest in resveratrol does not mean that the many other polyphenols present in abundance in red wine (such as anthocyanidins, proanthocyanidins, and phenolic acids) do not contribute to the properties of wine. Far from it! We have seen differently in Chapter 11 on p.117. However, the results obtained on the anticancer potential of resveratrol are so spectacular that this molecule has deserved and received particular attention in recent years.

WHAT IS RESVERATROL?

Resveratrol is a plant hormone isolated for the first time in 1940 from the roots of *Veratrum grandiflorum* (the name "resveratrol" comes from the Latin *res*, "thing," and *veratrum*, or "false hellebore," a plant belonging to the lily family). However, it was only in 1976 that its presence in grapevines was described. The production of resveratrol by grapevines is one of the plant's defense mechanisms against environmental

stress, such as pruning or attack by a microorganism such as the parasitic fungus *Botrytis cinerea* (which is responsible for gray-mold rot, or noble rot, in grapes). In general, grapevines located in regions with a more temperate and rainy climate are more susceptible to attack by microorganisms, and have in consequence higher levels of resveratrol than those growing in less hostile climates.

For example, a Pinot Noir from humid regions such as Burgundy or the Niagara Valley possesses high concentrations of resveratrol (10 mg per liter or more), since the very thin skin of this type of grape, coupled with its compact disposition in the center of each cluster, renders it particularly sensitive to attack by tiny fungi. The resveratrol produced by the plant in reaction to this attack is found almost exclusively in the skins and seeds of the grapes, which, as seen, explains its presence in red wine and its near-absence in white wine.

Resveratrol concentrations in red wine

As we noted earlier, there are relatively few dietary sources that supply significant amounts of resveratrol; the best source is unquestionably red wine, which has concentrations of up to 1 mg per 4-ounce (125-milliliter) glass of wine, depending on grape variety and the origin of the wine (see Table 18, p.150).

The large amount of resveratrol present in red wine is explained not only by the prolonged

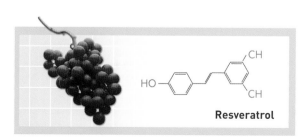

Resveratrol

fermentation period of the grape must (the grape juice that still contains the fruit's skins and seeds), during which the molecules are extracted from the skins and seeds, but also by the fact that the absence of oxygen in the bottle prevents the resveratrol from oxidizing. This is why raisins, which are also very rich in polyphenols, do not contain any resveratrol, which in their case is degraded by exposure to air and sunlight in the drying process.

Resveratrol content in various foods and beverages

Resveratrol is also found in large amounts in the grapes themselves. Unfortunately, its presence in the skins and seeds hinders its absorption into the body. Peanuts also look like they might be an adequate source of resveratrol, but their fat content means that the amount of peanuts a person would have to consume to obtain significant levels of resveratrol would result in an unhealthily high fat and calorie intake.

Grape juice also contains resveratrol, as does cranberry juice, but at levels that are ten times less than those in red wine. This difference is attributable to the long maceration process that the grape skins are subjected to, a process that allows a large quantity of resveratrol to be extracted from the skins. Resveratrol is extracted better from solutions containing alcohol, which again contributes to its increased concentration in red wine.

The hot pressing of grapes during the production of grape juice also allows the extraction of a non-negligible amount of resveratrol. Grape juice may thus represent an interesting alternative source of this molecule,

RESVERATROL CONTENT IN DIFFERENT FOODS AND BEVERAGES			
Food	**Resveratrol** (μg per 100 g)	**Beverage**	**Resveratrol** (μg per 125 ml)
Grapes	1500	Red wine	625*
Peanuts	150	White wine	38
Peanut butter	50	Grape juice	65
Blueberries	3	Cranberry juice	65
Raisins	0.01		

* Resveratrol concentration in red wine varies greatly from one grape variety to another and from one region to another, with values ranging from 1 to 13 mg per liter. Wine with a 5 mg per liter concentration, typical of Burgundies and Bordeaux, is used here as a reference. For white wine, values falling between 0.1 and 0.6 mg per liter are generally observed; we have chosen an average value of 0.3 mg per liter as an example. **Table 18**

especially for children who, because of their smaller total blood volume require a smaller intake to attain desirable levels of resveratrol. Grape juice is also suitable for pregnant and nursing women and anyone not wishing or unable to consume alcohol.

Grape juice for health

It is important to note that despite the relatively small amounts of resveratrol in grape juice, this beverage may nevertheless be very beneficial to health. Grape juice contains very high levels of anthocyanidins, phenolic acids, and other polyphenols which, as we have seen, have numerous antioxidant and chemopreventive properties. Like red and white wines, grape juice has significant amounts of piceid, a resveratrol derivative containing glucose in its structure. Scientists speculate that the degradation of this glucose by enzymes present in intestinal flora may release large quantities of resveratrol. Grape juice, in other words, is a star in its own right.

While its biological functions are still poorly understood, it is likely that this popular beverage will prove beneficial to children and adults alike.

Although it has not yet been clearly established that resveratrol is alone responsible for the beneficial effects of red wine on the rates of cardiovascular disease, many signs point to its playing a major role.

Other ways to get resveratrol

Resveratrol has been identified as the principal active ingredient in Ko-jo-kon, a traditional Asian remedy prepared from the ground-up roots of Japanese knotweed (*Polygonum cuspidatum*, also known as false bamboo), which has been used for thousands of years in Asia to treat cardiac, liver, and blood vessel ailments. The resveratrol currently sold in the West in the form of supplements is often an extract of this root preparation.

Chinese medicine also uses the roots of certain varieties of Veratrum to treat high blood pressure. In Ayurvedic tradition, an herbal remedy prepared principally from vine extracts, Darakchasava, has been used for millennia as a cardiac tonic. Given the omnipresence of wine in European and Mediterranean culture, it is rather ironic that the first clues as to the beneficial role played by resveratrol in disease prevention come once again from the East.

More interestingly, the societies in which wine is practically absent have still managed to identify and use preparations rich in resveratrol to treat cardiac and circulatory disorders. In our opinion, this example is a wonderful illustration of the concept that we described earlier: human curiosity and ingenuity cannot be underestimated when it comes to seeking remedies able to relieve illness, and a detailed study by modern science of traditional cuisines and medicines may lead to the identification of molecules that possess great benefits for health.

THE ANTICANCER PROPERTIES OF RESVERATROL

Although the anticancer potential of red wine remains to be more clearly established, there is no doubt that this anticancer activity is in large part due to the presence of resveratrol. In fact, of all naturally-occurring molecules possessing anticancer activity that have recently been studied, resveratrol commands a great deal of enthusiasm. In 1996, it was identified as the first molecule of dietary origin capable of interfering with the progression of cancer by inhibiting all three stages necessary for the development of the disease: initiation, promotion, and progression (**see Chapter 2, p.25**).

These early findings stimulated research on the mechanisms by which resveratrol acts on these processes. At the moment, the results we have are on the level of our expectations. Resveratrol has the capacity to interfere with several processes essential to the progression of tumors. Like curcumin (**see Chapter 9, p.99**), resveratrol is an extremely powerful anticancer molecule whose modes of action can be favorably compared to those of many drugs of synthetic origin that act to limit the growth of cancerous cells.

Current studies indicate that resveratrol is absorbed very rapidly into the body, meaning that the molecule reaches the bloodstream quickly and is on hand to act on cells. In models of animal cancers induced by chemical substances, resveratrol has proved very effective in preventing the development of breast, colon, and esophageal cancers. In some of these studies, resveratrol is administered orally in

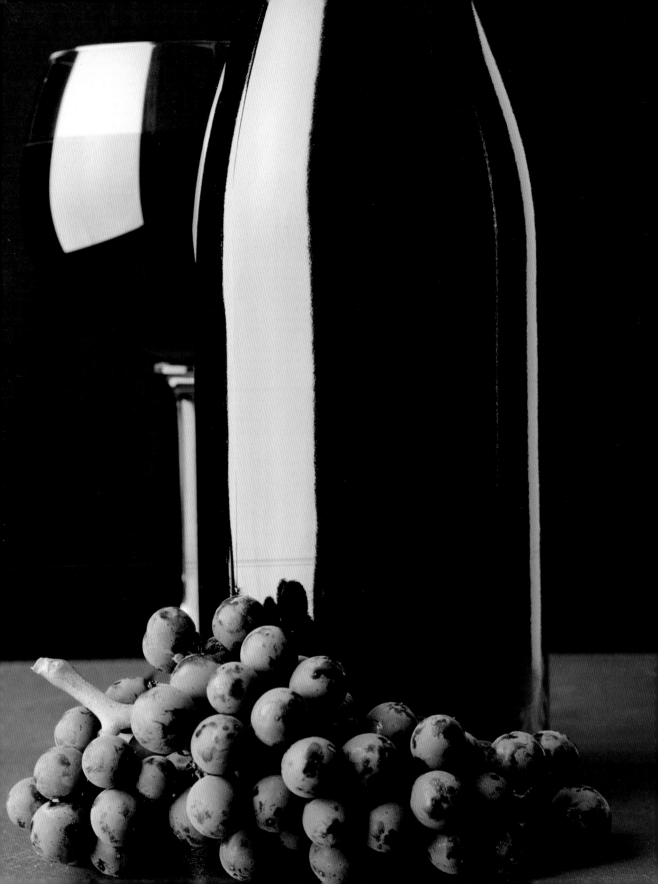

◀ **Drinking red wine** in moderation can help reduce the risk of developing both heart disease and cancer, two of the major health problems in the West.

small doses and its concentration in the blood varies from 0.1 to 2 micromoles per liter, an amount that may be attained in humans by the moderate consumption of red wine.

What resveratrol does in the body

In the course of its absorption, resveratrol goes through numerous structural modifications, but these changes probably do not alter in any way its anticancer properties. Piceatannol, one of the molecules produced by the degradation of the resveratrol molecule in the body, seems to be even more successful than its parent molecule at inducing the death of cancerous cells, such as leukemia or melanoma cells, at blood concentrations that are easily attainable by the consumption of red wine. These findings give cause for optimism on the effectiveness of resveratrol absorbed as food.

OTHER IMPORTANT FACTORS

We should remember that countries where wine consumption has been linked to lower mortality rates, particularly Mediterranean countries, are characterized by a diet rich in fruits, vegetables, legumes ,and nuts. These cuisines use olive oil as the principal source of fats use meat in only in moderation.

Studies on the anticancer potential of wine are still at a very early stage, but the observations made up until now are encouraging. As we have mentioned, red wine consumption seems to lower total mortality rates in a much more significant way than other types of alcohol. We believe that this effect is related to red wine's protective effect against cancer, which has not been observed for the consumption of other types of alcohol. Some data suggests that beer and spirit consumption, even in moderate amounts, may considerably increase the risk of several types of cancer. A Danish study indicated that the consumption of more than seven beers per week tripled the risk of mouth or esophageal cancer, while wine consumption halved the risk of developing these cancers. In the case of prostate cancer, a recent study showed that drinking one glass of wine per day causes a 40 percent decrease in the risk of developing this cancer, while the consumption of an equivalent amount of beer has no positive impact and may even slightly increase the risk of developing this disease.

In summary, if all types of alcohol may in moderate amounts reduce the risk of cardiovascular disease, this positive effect is to a certain extent counteracted by an increase in the risk of developing cancer in the case of alcoholic beverages other than wine. Up until now, the great majority of studies on the effect of alcohol on the development of cancer have been carried out without distinguishing between the types of alcohol consumed, which might explain why these studies generally conclude that alcohol consumption is a risk factor for cancer.

The studies in which the effect of wine was studied separately from that of other types of alcohol indicate not only that wine consumption does not cause cancer, but that on the contrary, it may reduce the incidence of several cancers. Although additional studies are certainly needed to confirm the anticancer potential associated with wine, the data currently available, as well as the beneficial effect of wine-drinking on longevity, indicate the importance of drinking wine to maintain good health.

In the context of a strategy of cancer prevention through diet, it is clear that the moderate consumption of red wine alone should be considered, since this alcohol does more than reduce the risk of cardiovascular disease. It is unique in having a positive impact on the decrease in risk for cancer.

LONG LIVE RESVERATROL!

A particularly dynamic field of resveratrol research concerns the ability of this molecule to increase longevity. It has been known for some time that limiting caloric intake is the best way of increasing longevity in living organisms. For example, laboratory rats put on a strict diet live 30 percent longer than rats that are allowed to eat at will. This effect may be related to the activation of a family of proteins known as sirtuins, which are thought to lengthen cell life by giving cells the necessary time to repair the DNA damage that occurs as they age.

Even more interesting from a nutritional point of view are recent results indicating that certain molecules of dietary origin, including quercetin and especially resveratrol, are very powerful sirtuin activators. It is this activation that may increase cell longevity. For example, the addition of resveratrol to a growth culture of single-celled organisms such as yeast increases cell lifespan by 80 percent. Generally, yeasts live for 19 generations, but adding resveratrol boosted life expectancy to a maximum of 38 generations!

The same tendency was observed for more complex organisms. Adding resveratrol to the diet of worms and fruit flies caused an increase in lifespan on the order of 15 percent for worms and 29 percent for fruit flies. Resveratrol may thus have the capacity to activate the cell's repair mechanisms and lengthen life by imitating, to a certain extent, the effect of restricting calorie intake.

Could the lower mortality rates observed in populations that regularly consume red wine in moderate amounts be related to a lengthening of cell life due to resveratrol? We cannot yet say. However, one thing is certain: with its beneficial effects on the cardiovascular system and the protection it affords against the development of cancer as well as its capacity to lengthen cell life, resveratrol is probably one of the molecules of dietary origin that offers the greatest benefits for human health.

NOTHING IN EXCESS

By including red wine in the list of foods that may help prevent cancer, our intention is not to trivialize all manner of alcohol consumption. Red wine or no red wine, excessive alcohol consumption is harmful to health, whether because of an increased risk of cardiac disease and cancer, or because of the host of serious social problems that are aggravated by alcohol abuse, from highway accident mortality to domestic violence.

However, numerous scientific findings support the diverse benefits associated with the moderate consumption of red wine. Although resveratrol is certainly not the only substance responsible for the positive effects on cardiovascular health seen with red wine, it seems that this molecule bears the greatest responsibility for the anticancer properties of red wine.

Thus we can recommend drinking red wine. It truly is the best source of resveratrol currently available. Most people who drink alcohol do so in moderation, and they may benefit from the "side effects" of moderate consumption: the prevention of chronic diseases such as cancer and cardiovascular disease. On a more congenial note, red wine is often accompanied by good food, shared in an atmosphere that reduces stress. To be effective, red wine should be drunk in moderation as part of a balanced diet.

In summary

- **Red wine** is truly a unique alcoholic beverage. This is because it contains a great variety of phytochemical compounds that offer several significant health benefits.

- **The resveratrol present** in red wine possesses powerful anticancer activity, which may be responsible for the beneficial effects of wine on the prevention of certain cancers.

- **The moderate** consumption of red wine as part of a balanced diet is a simple and pleasant way of helping prevent the development of cancer.

"Love chocolate completely, without complexes or false shame; remember, 'There is no reasonable man without a spark of madness.'"

François de La Rochefoucauld (1613–1680)

Chocolate: a Good Obsession

It might seem unbelievable, but it's true – good-quality, dark chocolate in moderate amounts is actually good for you! The early Mexicans used the beans as money and Linnaeus named chocolate "the food of the gods." Chocolate deserves its reputation, being rich in important polyphenols.

The cacao tree was in all likelihood first domesticated by the Mayas, who cultivated it at least 3000 years ago in the Yucatan region of Mexico, although it probably originated in the Amazon and Orenoque basins. The Mayas and their successors, the Toltecs and especially the Aztecs, attached great importance to the beans harvested from this tree, which they used both as legal currency and in the preparation of a bitter spiced drink, *xocoatl*. For the Aztecs, the *cacahuaquahuilt*, or cacao tree, was a gift from Quetzalcóatl, the god represented by a feathered serpent who, according to legend, was to return one day, recovering his kingdom and bringing the Aztecs all the treasure of Paradise.

When Hernan Cortés (1485-1547) landed on the Mexican coast, near present-day Tabasco, in April 1519, the Aztec emperor Montezuma II was convinced that the Spaniard was the descendant of Quetzalcóatl. The explorer was greeted as a god. He was offered gold, plantations… and chocolate, drunk from a goblet of encrusted gold. Cortés, however, was more drawn to the riches of Aztec civilization than to chocolate, installing himself as ruler, taking the emperor hostage and conquering Tenochtitlán (Mexico City), the capital of the empire, in August 1521. It was the end of the Aztec civilization but only the beginning of the invasion of the world by chocolate. The first cargoes of cacao beans arrived in Spain in 1582, the beans quickly gaining widespread acceptance.

The *xocoatl* consumed by the peoples of Central America was very different from the chocolate we know today. The beans were roasted and ground to extract a pasty mass, to which was added water and various spices, notably pepper, pimento, and cinnamon. The mass was heated, causing the butter to rise to the surface, and then the substance was beaten to obtain a thick, foamy liquid that was drunk cold. The word "chocolate" itself actually refers to the sound made by the whisk as it helped dissolve and then whip up the liquid: *xoco* ("noise") and *atl* ("water").

The Europeans adopted this procedure, but soon replaced the spices with sugar to reduce the bitterness of this otherwise refreshing drink. Chocolate thus acquired the "divine" taste that helped it spread throughout Europe. It was a beverage unique in its power to seduce and its capacity to incite cravings and inflame passions. In 1753, when Carl Linnaeus needed a Latin name for the cacao tree, he came up with *Theobroma cacao*, which literally means "food of the gods." There were no objections recorded!

THE PHYTOCHEMICAL COMPOUNDS IN CHOCOLATE

Cacao beans are composed of 50–57 percent fat. True, these lipids are mostly saturated: 35 percent stearic acid and 25 percent palmitic acid. However, a good proportion (35 percent) is oleic acid, a monounsaturated fatty acid found primarily in olive oil and known to have positive effects on cardiovascular system health. Chocolate's principal lipid, stearic acid, is only weakly absorbed into the body, where it is partially (about 15 percent) transformed into oleic acid by the liver. Thus dark chocolate is food that can be described as neutral as to its impact on blood cholesterol.

The case of milk chocolate is different. A significant portion of the lipid content in milk chocolate comes from milk fats, as well as some vegetable fats used in candy as filler. Despite its high sugar content, dark chocolate has a relatively low glycemic index, half that of white bread and similar to that of orange juice. All in all, the high fat and sugar content of both types of chocolate makes for a calorie-rich food that should be eaten in moderation.

The interest in the potential health benefits of chocolate did not come about as a result of its fat and sugar content! Chocolate contains an abundance of polyphenols; a small square of dark chocolate has twice the polyphenol content of a glass of red wine and about as much as a cup of green tea brewed for the correct length of time (**see Table 19, left**).

The principal polyphenols found in cacao are the same as those present in large quantities in green tea, the catechins. Proanthocyanidins, the polymers, or long chains, formed by these molecules, make up between 12 and 48 percent of the weight of the cacao bean. Proanthocyanidins are renowned as powerful antioxidants (**see Chapter 11, p.123**), so it is not surprising that chocolate possesses similar properties. In fact, according to recent analyses, chocolate, and especially dark chocolate, possesses truly sensational antioxidant activity.

RICH IN POLYPHENOLS!	
Source	**Polyphenol content** (mg)*
Dark chocolate (50 g)	300
Green tea	250
Cacao (2 teaspoons)	200
Red wine (125 ml)	150
Milk chocolate (50 g)	100

* Polyphenol content may vary significantly depending on provenance and preparation method.

Table 19

THE MANUFACTURE OF CHOCOLATE

After a short fermentation period, cacao beans are dried and roasted at high temperature to develop their flavor and aroma. The beans are then broken into pieces to remove their shells, and ground until a thick liquid that solidifies at room temperature, the cocoa mass, is obtained. This substance may be used as is in the preparation of chocolate, or it can be pressed to extract a large part of its fat content, which is the cocoa butter.

How different kinds of chocolate are made
Cocoa powder is made by pulverizing the cocoa mass and then removing the cocoa butter. Dark chocolate is the product of a mixture of cocoa mass and added sugar and cocoa butter. The amount of cocoa mass used is generally between 35 and 70 percent of the content of the final product. If it is more than 70 percent, the chocolate is bitter to taste, finding use mostly as cooking chocolate. The same technique is used to make milk chocolate, except that milk solids are added, thus reducing the cocoa mass content to about 20-40 percent.

Real chocolate versus chocolate candy
Fine dark and milk chocolates have little in common with the products consumed in large quantities by North Americans, which are more chocolate-flavored candy than chocolate. These products contain very little cocoa (federal laws prohibit their being labeled "chocolate"). Instead of cocoa butter, they contain fillers, such as saturated fats. This is why "chocolate" candy, which contains more fats and sugar than does dark chocolate, is a source of cholesterol.

One cup of hot chocolate generates antioxidant activity that is five times greater than that of a cup of black tea, three times greater than that of green tea, and twice as strong as a glass of red wine. It is now believed that this high polyphenol content is the primary factor responsible for the positive health benefits of chocolate.

THE BENEFICIAL EFFECTS OF CHOCOLATE
In its New World beginnings, chocolate was favored as a food that relieved the effects of fatigue. Legend has it that the emperor Montezuma could drink up to fifty goblets of *xocoatl* per day, which may seem enormous, but was probably the amount he needed for support in the day's tasks (he kept a harem of 600 concubines). This historical anecdote is the source of the many beliefs in the aphrodisiac virtues of chocolate, which, incidentally, still remain to be proven.

Over the course of history, chocolate has been regarded as not only a food pleasant to the taste, but also as a remedy for different ailments, especially angina and circulatory problems. This positive association of chocolate and health lasted until the end of the 19th century; it was only with the industrialization of chocolate production and the manufacture of sugar-filled candies containing very little cacao (and fewer polyphenols) that chocolate began to be perceived as a substance harmful to health.

Up until now, researchers have studied mostly the potential impact of chocolate on cardiovascular disease in populations that consume large quantities of cacao. For example, the Kuna, a tribe from the San Blass archipelago off the coast of Panama, are great eaters of cacao, which they consume as a drink prepared in a way similar to that of the Aztecs. The Kuna drink about five cups of cacao per day, and even more in several cases, and

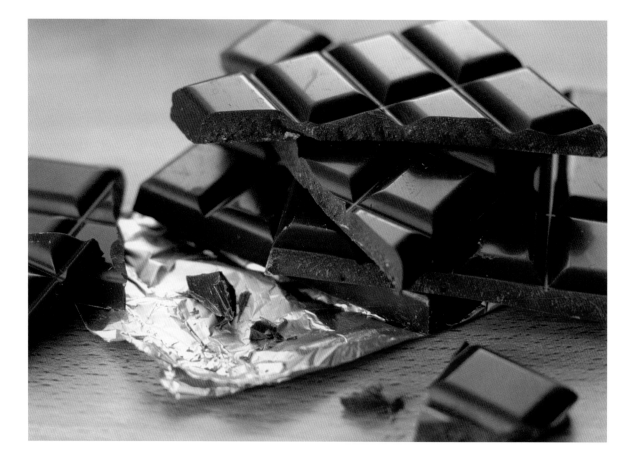

▲ **High-quality dark chocolate** is not only an enjoyable treat, but also contains phytochemicals that may help prevent the development of cancer.

also use cacao as an ingredient in other dishes. Interest in the Kuna lies in the fact that although they have a diet heavy in salt, their blood pressure is unusually low. This characteristic does not seem to be genetic in origin, since tribe members who leave the islands to live elsewhere experience an increase in blood pressure.

Cacao's beneficial effect on the cardiovascular system may be related to its antioxidant activity. The ingestion of moderate quantities of cacao causes the blood's antioxidant capacity to rise, thus diminishing the oxidation of proteins

responsible for the formation of atheromatous plaques (plaques that protrude into blood vessels and block blood flow). However, we should note that this effect disappears when chocolate is eaten together with milk, because of a dramatic change in polyphenol absorption.

Another effect of chocolate that certainly contributes to its benefits for the cardiovascular system is the reduction of harmful blood platelet activity, which reduces the risk of clot formation.

CHOCOLATE: AN ANTICANCER FOOD?
The similarity of the phytochemical content in cacao and that of other foods suspected of playing a role in cancer prevention allows us to imagine that cacao may also exhibit some

CHOCOLATE: A GOOD OBSESSION **161**

anticancer properties. Although studies on the capacity of the polyphenols in chocolate to prevent cancer are only beginning, the results so far are encouraging.

Scientists have observed that the proanthocyanidins in cocoa mass are able to slow the development of certain cancers, especially lung cancer, induced in laboratory animals. The absorption of the polyphenols in cacao may cause a sharp drop in the levels of EGFR, a receptor essential to angiogenesis and the growth of cancerous cells. Just like the proanthocyanidins present in cranberries (**see Chapter 11, p.123**), the proanthocyanidins in cacao may contribute to the prevention of cancer by acting on the multiple events involved in the progression of this disease. Further studies are needed to establish chocolate's anticancer potential with greater certainty, but current findings are very positive and certainly do not justify the bad reputation that chocolate has acquired over the last few decades.

How much is enough?
The daily consumption of 1½ ounces (40 grams) of dark chocolate (chocolate containing 70 percent cocoa mass) may supply the body with a significant dose of polyphenols, and thus confer health benefits for the prevention of cardiovascular disease and cancer. The preventive effect will be enhanced if dark chocolate consumption replaces or reduces the amount of the sugary and fat-filled foods consumed. These snacks contain no anticancer compounds, and eating them causes blood cholesterol levels to rise and

leads, among other things, to weight gain. In other words, if we admit that sugar intake will always be an important part of human dietary habits because of the pleasurable feeling it induces, changing these habits so as to substitute dark chocolate for sugar-filled junk food with no nutritional benefits may have a significant impact on the prevention of chronic diseases such as cancer. Who said that healthy eating couldn't be enjoyable?

In summary

● **Dark chocolate,** which contains 70 percent cocoa mass, supplies the body with important amounts of polyphenols that are potentially capable of exercising beneficial effects on some chronic illnesses, including cancer and cardiovascular disease.

● **The daily consumption** of 1½ ounces (40 grams) of chocolate that is 70 percent cocoa mass may have definite health benefits and should replace or reduce that of sugar- and fat-filled candies that lack any phytochemical content.

part 3

day-to-day Nutrition Therapy

- Supplements: Friend or Foe?

- On Today's Menu: Fighting Cancer!

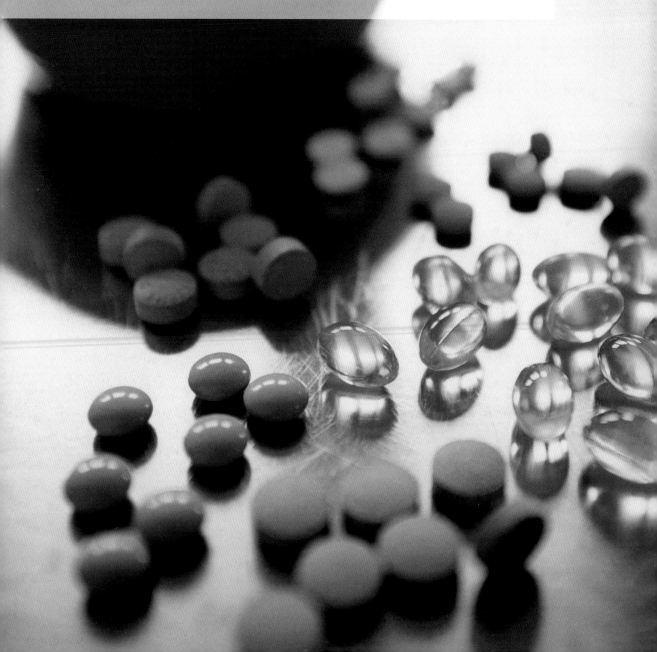

"All substances are poisons; there is none which is not a poison. The right dose differentiates a poison from a remedy."

Paracelsus (1493–1541)

17

Supplements: Friend or Foe?

In today's fast-moving world, people are more and more inclined to take a few vitamin pills and think that it makes up for the lack of a healthy diet. The research behind this book shows that the truth is very different, and that nothing can substitute for a balanced diet made up of fresh, whole foods.

Some people will always be tempted to look for the shortcut. If such people become aware of the essential role played by phytochemical compounds in cancer prevention, their first reflex might not necessarily be to choose to modify their eating habits to include foods that constitute good sources of these molecules. Instead, they might try to find out if these molecules are available as food supplements!

In the West, we have made a virtual cult of food supplements, so that many people now prefer taking vitamin C pills to eating oranges. To put it simply, this situation is completely absurd. We live in a time of unprecedented abundance. Fresh fruits and vegetables may be easily obtained all year round at very reasonable prices. In spite of this great wealth, fruit and vegetable consumption remains relatively very

low everywhere in the West, while sales of vitamin supplements are skyrocketing. In 2004, they reached 20.3 billion dollars in the United States alone. Supplements seem well on their way to becoming an essential component of today's diet, but sadly, at the expense of fruits and vegetables.

This is a regrettable situation. Recent findings have established an important point: the many health benefits that may be attributed to the consumption of fruits and vegetables cannot be explained solely by their vitamin content. In fact, in the case of cancer prevention, the subject that interests us, vitamins play only a very minor role, much smaller than that played by phytochemical compounds.

Unsurprisingly, the pharmaceutical industry has already reacted to this news by isolating the principal active phytochemical compounds and marketing them in the form of supplements. An incredible number of products containing some of the molecules described in this book already exist: ellagic acid, curcumin, anthocyanidins, proanthocyanidins, isoflavones, I3C, and sulforaphane may all be easily purchased over the Internet, where they are promoted and sold on the premise that they reduce cancer risk.

Attempting to describe the health-enhancing properties of fruits and vegetables in terms of a single phytochemical compound is not only reductive, but illogical. Broccoli cannot be reduced to its sulforaphane content, any more than we can consider that the health benefits of raspberries are due only to the presence of ellagic acid. Plants have developed at least 20,000 of these compounds to defend themselves and maintain good health, and it is certain that every one of them has some role to play in preserving plant cell equilibrium. If you choose to adopt the foods we have discussed here, even a simple meal may supply you with thousands of phytochemical compounds. It would be counterproductive to replace dietary sources that are as fundamental as fruits and vegetables by molecules in pill or capsule form.

Beyond these slightly philosophical considerations, and excepting the obvious financial ones, some good practical reasons exist for avoiding synthetically manufactured pills, especially in the case of phytochemical compound supplements.

1. Effectiveness

The use of supplements is generally based on the idea that if a given molecule has specific health benefits, a higher dose of this molecule will provide even greater benefits. This is totally untrue! In many cases, and especially in that of soy, what occurs is exactly the opposite. The active compound in the food is less beneficial, and may even be dangerous, when it is administered in an isolated manner, outside the context of the whole food.

2. Diversity

Eating the whole food provides greater benefits than taking supplements that contain only one of the food's constituent parts, because of the presence of numerous phytochemical compounds in that food. Any food's effectiveness against cancer is increased when specific processes involved in the growth of cancer are targeted by the combined efforts of all the molecules present, something that is impossible to achieve by taking a supplement based upon a single molecule (see **Figure 31**, left).

ADVANTAGES OF FOODS VS. FOOD SUPPLEMENTS

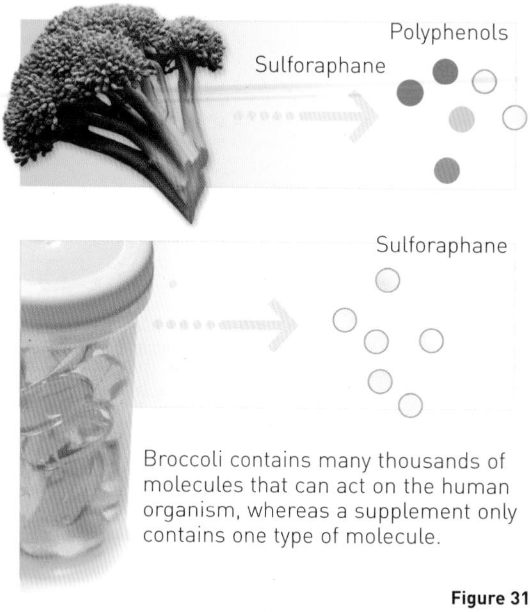

Polyphenols
Sulforaphane

Sulforaphane

Broccoli contains many thousands of molecules that can act on the human organism, whereas a supplement only contains one type of molecule.

Figure 31

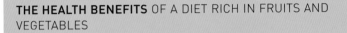

THE HEALTH BENEFITS OF A DIET RICH IN FRUITS AND VEGETABLES

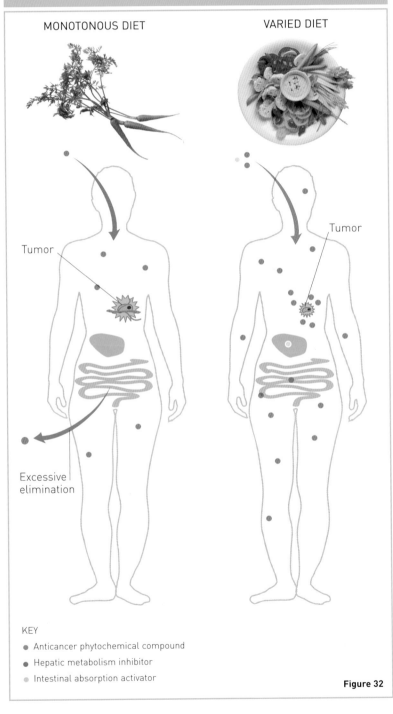

MONOTONOUS DIET

VARIED DIET

Tumor

Tumor

Excessive elimination

KEY

• Anticancer phytochemical compound
• Hepatic metabolism inhibitor
• Intestinal absorption activator

Figure 32

For example, cruciferous vegetables contain molecules that act to accelerate the detoxification of carcinogenic substances, but they also contain many other phytochemical compounds, notably polyphenols. Thus it is premature to reduce their anticancer properties to this detoxification process alone.

Not only does the use of supplements not provide the health benefits associated with the entire arsenal of molecules naturally present in foods, but the presence of large quantities of these same molecules in the form of supplements may render the absorption of other healthful compounds less effective. In fact, overloading the absorption systems at the intestinal wall causes these systems to become less effective at recognizing the different compounds supplied by food, which leads to weaker absorption of these molecules into the bloodstream.

This drop in the absorption of certain molecules associated with foods is far from trivial; it may be responsible for lowering the ability of anticancer compounds to accomplish their tasks effectively. A large number of the molecules present in foods are able to act on an

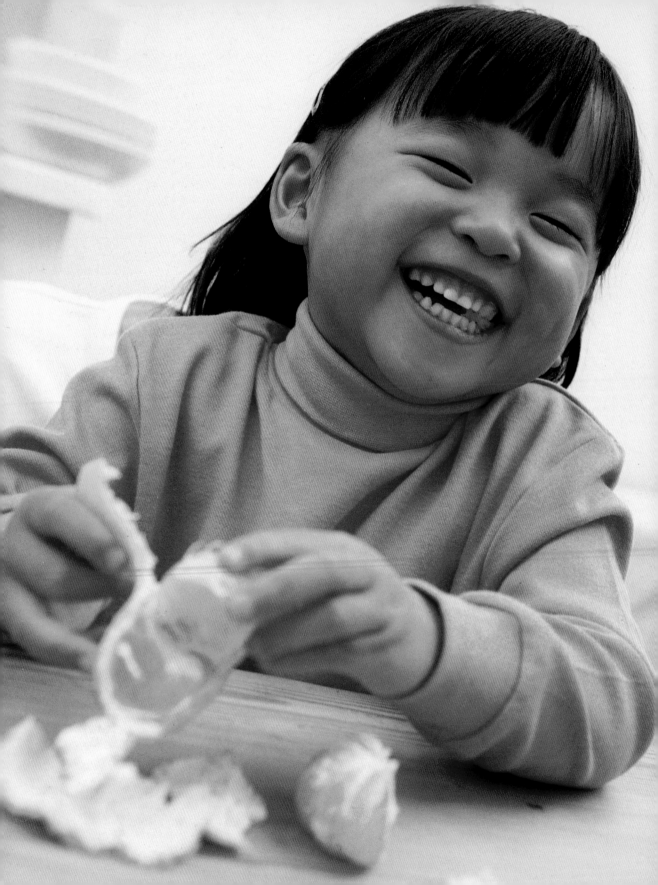

organism's metabolism. Therefore, their absorption has important repercussions on the quantity of anticancer molecules present in the bloodstream (see Figure 32, p.167). For example, certain molecules lower the metabolism of foreign substances by the liver, while others act on the intestines, reducing the degradation or increasing the absorption of phytochemical compounds. In both cases, the result is similar: the time spent by these anticancer compounds in the body before being eliminated is increased, thus boosting their anticancer activity.

3. Quality

It is also important to understand that many supplements do not contain the quantities of molecules that one would normally find in the whole foods. Without necessarily doubting the word, or at the very least, the printed claims, of manufacturers, it must be remembered that the great majority of phytochemical compounds are very reactive molecules and they are thus necessarily unstable.

There are many examples of the effect this instability can have on the content of a supplement. One of the most spectacular is the case of resveratrol. Analyses conducted by independent laboratories showed that the quantity of resveratrol present in the capsules studied was so small that a person would have to consume thousands of them just to ingest the equivalent of the resveratrol contained in a single glass of wine. At today's prices, this means that the necessary dose of resveratrol would cost, in supplements, the equivalent of a glass of wine from a $2,000 bottle!

Naturally occurring phytoprotective elements are generally always well protected from degradation inside the cellular compartments of the plants that contain them. When these compartments are extracted, the molecules are exposed to air and to degradation enzymes and are destroyed, either by oxidation or enzymatic degradation. This means that these molecules should be consumed in the form that most closely resembles their original plant forms. Industrially made preparations in which the fruit or vegetable has been processed beyond recognition should be rejected.

For example, if you wish to use flax seeds as a source of omega-3 fatty acids, avoid buying seeds that have already been ground. Instead, try to purchase the whole seeds that you can then grind at home, thus preserving the integrity of the essential lipids present. For the same reason, avoid using flax seed oil. Even though the oil is an important source of these lipids, the great sensitivity of polyunsaturated omega-3s to the oxygen in air causes a rapid degradation that will prevent you from enjoying the health benefits provided by these molecules.

DOES ANYONE NEED SUPPLEMENTS?

In summary, if a person's diet lacks vitamins, minerals, and anticancer compounds because he or she does not consume sufficient quantities of fruits and vegetables, the solution to the problem lies not in taking supplements, but in making profound, far-reaching changes to diet. There are no, and there will be no, miracle cures that are able to entirely repair the damage caused by a diet of poor quality. You cannot eat just anything and get off the hook by taking a pill!

◄ **Eating whole foods,** instead of taking supplements, allows the body to benefit from the wide range of chemical compounds they contain.

"The destiny of nations depends on the manner in which they feed themselves."

Jean Anthelme Brillat-Savarin, *The Physiology of Taste* (1825)

18

On Today's Menu: Fighting Cancer!

There are many simple and practical lifestyle changes that you can make to help reduce your chance of developing cancer. Among the most important are quitting smoking and getting regular exercise, and, of course, eating a varied diet rich in the foods described in the previous chapters.

CHANGING YOUR LIFESTYLE TO HELP PREVENT CANCER

We would like to conclude by offering some suggestions on changes that can be made in the lifestyle now in vogue in our society, changes that truly have the potential to decrease your risk of being stricken by cancer.

We have seen that the principal characteristic of the Western diet is its extremity, in its excesses as well as in what it lacks – there is too much sugar and there are too many fats and too many red meats, on the one hand, and too few fruits and vegetables and too little dietary fiber, on the other. Reestablishing a balance in dietary intake between these two extremes while avoiding selected "bad" foods as much as possible (see Figure 33, p.172) can only have beneficial consequences on the prevention of chronic diseases such as cancer. But changes in diet, however essential, form only part of a bigger picture. Other changes in lifestyle, described below, may also have an enormous impact on the risk of being affected by cancer.

Quit smoking

Given that one-third of all cancers are directly related to tobacco use, it goes without saying that quitting smoking is one of the lifestyle changes that can have the greatest impact on cancer prevention. The list of harmful effects associated with tobacco use is a very long one: a thirty-fold increase in the risk of lung cancer, a significant increase in the risk of cancers of the mouth and throat and of the pancreas and bladder, and a staggering increase in the risk of being affected by fatal cardiovascular disease, not to mention the many unpleasant side effects smokers put up with, such as loss of smell and taste, chronic fatigue, and so on.

Happily, society has taken giant steps in controlling tobacco use. These include intensive information campaigns stressing the dangers of tobacco use and an ever greater number of public spaces where smoking is forbidden, as well as the heady increases in the cost of tobacco. All of these efforts have brought about a significant reduction in the proportion of smokers in our society as a direct consequence.

Even the most hardened smokers today admit that tobacco use is harmful to health, and most of them express their desire to kick the habit. These people should not feel any shame or embarrassment if they find it difficult to quit. Nicotine is one of the most powerful drugs found in nature and creates a dependence that is extremely difficult to overcome. However, because this drug continues to be sold freely, its use cannot be effectively curbed and all efforts must instead be funneled into informing people about its toxic nature.

We can only encourage smokers who wish to stop smoking to use all of the means presently at their disposal to help them to put an end to their dependency. Quitting smoking is the one decision that will have by far the greatest impact on your quality of life.

Lower your calorie intake

Avoid buying industrially prepared and processed foods, whether as snacks or as main meals. These products contain far too much sugar, harmful fats, and salt and, compared to fresh foods, are poor in nutritive elements. Reclaim your kitchen and your cooking. You will be able to better control the quantity and quality of the ingredients that make up your diet. Instead of replacing butter with margarine, use olive oil as much as possible as a source of dietary fat. You will benefit from its healthful fats knowing that it also possesses anticancer properties of its own.

Finally, a simple way of reducing your calorie intake is to consider hamburgers, hotdogs, French fries, potato chips, and soft drinks as occasional treats rather than foods that can or should be eaten on a daily basis. Like all animals, human beings are strongly attracted to foods rich in fats and sugar, because the consumption of such food induces a feeling of real pleasure that incites us to repeat the act. It is pointless to repress this instinct completely, but you can turn the situation to your advantage by consuming these foods only occasionally. You will then be able to fully satisfy your cravings without experiencing the health problems associated with a surplus of calories, or a bad conscience!

Reduce red meat consumption

A diet rich in red meats (beef, lamb, and pork) considerably increases the risk of colon cancer, and also supplies huge amounts of calories in the form of fats that may contribute to excess weight. Try to vary your daily menus by using leaner meats, such as chicken or fish (ideally, fish

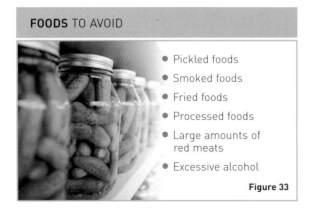

FOODS TO AVOID

- Pickled foods
- Smoked foods
- Fried foods
- Processed foods
- Large amounts of red meats
- Excessive alcohol

Figure 33

that are rich in omega-3 fatty acids), occasionally replacing your daily serving of meat by other sources of protein, such as legumes. Eating is not synonymous with eating meat!

A good way to decrease meat consumption is to reconsider the place it occupies in daily meals. Meat does not necessarily need to be front and center in a dish or a meal for us to enjoy its taste. For example, North African couscous and various sautéed Asian stir-fries are delicious examples of meat used as accompaniment to dishes based on grains and vegetables.

Avoid foods containing potentially cancer-causing substances

Smoked meats and other foods containing preservatives such as nitrites (bacon, sausages, prepared delicatessen meats, ham, and so forth) increase the risk of certain cancers because the nitrites present are transformed through body chemistry into very carcinogenic substances.

Limit the consumption of these foods as much as possible, avoiding barbecued meats as well. When meat is cooked over a flame, the greasy drippings that fall and catch fire produce toxic substances known as aromatic hydrocarbons, which rise to adhere to the surface of the meat and may act as carcinogens.

Other cancer-causing substances known as heterocyclic amines are also formed by cooking animal proteins at high temperatures. However, recent studies suggest that marinating the meat in the presence of acids such as lemon juice may reduce the formation of these toxins.

Avoid foods using salt a preservative. Countries where large quantities of salted or pickled foods are consumed (such as Portugal, Japan, China, and Latin America) have high incidences of stomach cancer, often associated with a high intake of heavily salted foods.

Exercise regularly

Regular exercise is an excellent habit that helps maintain overall fitness and muscle tone. Recent findings now suggest a relationship between physical activity and a reduced risk of certain cancers, such as breast and colon cancers.

Of course, regular physical activity reduces obesity, an important factor that increases the risk of cancer. Another study indicates that moderate physical activity (three to five hours of walking per week, for example) significantly reduces the risk of mortality in women diagnosed with breast cancer. It is not necessary to undertake an Olympic-caliber training program to enjoy the health benefits of exercise: walk as much and as often as you can during the day. Using the stairs at your place of work instead of the elevator is a good way to start.

AN OPTIMAL CANCER PREVENTION DIET

A close relationship exists between the nature of diet and the risks of developing several types of cancers. We can use our knowledge about this relationship to effect important changes in lifestyle, thereby preventing cancer at the source, before it becomes too formidable an enemy.

It is important to grasp that none of the foods described in this book are in and of themselves miracle cures for cancer. The very concept of "miracle cure," so popular and pervasive in society, is responsible for the lack of interest shown by people in the impact of their own lifestyle choices on the development of serious diseases such as cancer. We believe that cancer should be approached in a more realistic manner, by admitting that even given our current scientific and medical knowledge, this disease is too often a fatal one, one that we must do everything in our power to fight with the tools at our disposal. We should be afraid of

FOODS THAT FIGHT CANCER:
A POCKET GUIDE

Food	Serving size
Brussels sprouts	½ cup (uncooked)
Broccoli, cauliflower, cabbage	½ cup (uncooked)
Garlic	2 cloves
Onions, shallots	½ cup (uncooked)
Spinach, watercress	½ cup (uncooked)
Freshly ground flax seeds	½ cup
Tomato paste	1 tablespoon
Turmeric	1 tablespoon
Black pepper	½ teaspoon
Blueberries, raspberries, blackberries	½ cup (fresh)
Dried cranberries	½ cup
Grapes	½ cup
Dark chocolate (70% cacao)	1 ½ oz
Citrus fruit juice	½ cup
Green tea	3 times 8 oz
Red wine	1 glass

Table 20

cancer – however, instead of paralyzing us or invading our thoughts obsessively, this fear should be constructive, pushing us to adopt the behaviors that are most likely to counter the disease in the first place. In the same way that a person chooses to control her fear of fire by installing a smoke detector in every room in her house, our fear of cancer might incite us to react by modifying our lifestyles, and especially our diets, in order to protect ourselves from this disease as best we can.

Once again, cancer prevention is made possible by changes in diet, such as including foods that constitute abundant sources of anticancer compounds. By referring to all the available scientific data on the anticancer potential of compounds of dietary origin, we can put together what may be called an optimal cancer prevention diet, which is a diet based in large part on the daily intake of foods known to be exceptional sources of anticancer molecules (see Table 20, left).

The following recommendations are based on the concepts we have described in this book.

Variety is the spice of life
The presence of different classes of anticancer molecules prevents the development of cancer by interfering with specific processes involved in the progression of this disease. No one food contains all of the anticancer molecules able to act on these processes as a whole (see Table 21, opposite), and this is why incorporating the greatest possible variety of foods into diet is so important. For example, eating cruciferous vegetables, as well as vegetables belonging to the garlic family, helps the body eliminate carcinogenic substances, thus reducing the ability of these substances to cause mutations in DNA that may lead to cancerous cells.

In the same vein, the absorption of green tea, berries, and soy prevents the formation of the new blood vessels necessary for microtumor growth. The microtumors remain blocked at a latent stage of development. Certain molecules associated with these foods are able to act on more than one stage of cancer, thus maximizing the protection afforded by diet. We have only to think of the resveratrol in grapes, which can act on all three stages of cancer. There is also the genistein in soy, which, in addition to being a phytoestrogen that weakens the sometimes harmful effects of sex hormones, is also a powerful inhibitor of several proteins involved in uncontrolled cancer cell growth.

This diversity of anticancer molecules in food is crucial because cancer cells can exploit many different pathways in order to grow. It is misguided to attempt to control their talent at bypassing obstacles by using anticancer molecules that only interfere with a single process. A simple analogy is useful here: if you are trying to carry a bucket of water that is full of holes, stopping up only some of the holes will not get you very far; you will have to plug them all up. It is the same for cancer: an attack has to be carried out on several fronts before we can hope to succeed in preventing the disease from getting out of control and attaining its frightening maturity.

Eat moderately and regularly

The daily absorption of anticancer phytochemical compounds is a wonderful example of metronomic therapy, in which the continuous administration of anticancer molecules keeps precancerous cells in disequilibrium by preventing their growth.

This concept of continuous combat is an important one, because cancer must be

---

A PREVENTION DIET:
FRUITS AND VEGETABLES

- Increase consumption
- Vary consumption
- Choose dishes that are made from several varieties of fruits and vegetables
- Eat fruits and vegetables every day

PRINCIPAL ACTIVITY SITES OF ANTICANCER COMPOUNDS PRESENT IN DIET (FOOD)

Goals targeted by nutraceuticals	Green tea	Turmeric	Soy	Cruciferous vegetables	Garlic and onions	Grapes and berries	Citrus fruits	Tomatoes	Omega-3s	Dark chocolate
Reduction of carcinogenic potential				●	●	●	●			
Inhibition of tumoral cell growth	●	●	●	●	●	●	●	●	●	●
Induction of tumoral cell death		●	●	●	●	●	●			
Interference with angiogenesis	●	●	●				●		●	
Impact on the immune system		●				●			●	

Table 21

THE TREATMENT OF CANCER WITH ANTICANCER COMPOUNDS PRESENT IN FOOD

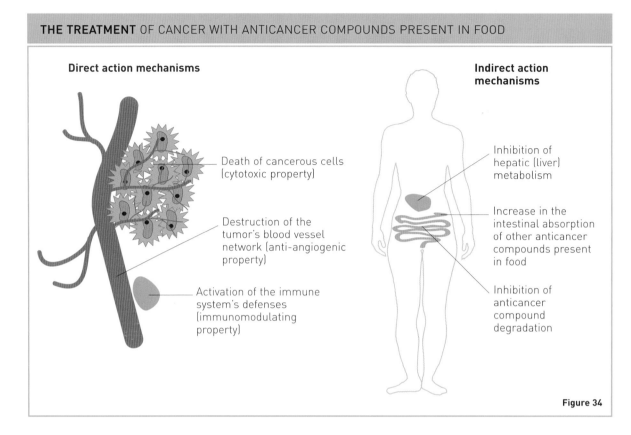

Figure 34

considered a chronic disease that requires constant treatment to keep it in a latent state. In other words, there is no point in eating one extravagant meal containing enormous amounts of the foods described here on a Sunday and then ignoring these recommendations and eating poorly for the remainder of the week. This way of thinking, and eating, does not contribute anything to cancer prevention efforts, any more than a single massive dose of insulin will allow a person with diabetes to solve his or her glycemic problems over the long term.

It is often said that moderation is the key to a healthy diet, and the same is true for cancer prevention. Preventing cancer through diet must be seen as constant, moderate work, made possible by a decision to make lifestyle changes.

Effective eating

We have seen that the anticancer agents present in food are often capable of acting directly on a tumor and restricting its development by causing the death of cancerous cells and by preventing the tumor from progressing to a more advanced stage. For example, an anticancer agent may work by interfering with the formation of a new blood vessel network or by stimulating the response of the body's immune system (**see Figure 34, above**).

If one specific type of anticancer molecule is capable of such activity, what might a combination of several different types of molecules accomplish? Researchers have found that combining foods with distinct anticancer compounds allows them to target different processes involved in tumor growth, as well as making their activity more effective. Thanks to this synergy, a molecule's anticancer activity may be considerably enhanced by the presence of another molecule; this is a very important property of compounds found in food that are generally present in small quantities in the bloodstream. For example, neither curcumin nor the principal polyphenol present in green tea, EGCG, are capable of inducing cell death by themselves when each is present in small quantities. However, when these two molecules are added simultaneously to a cancer cell culture, they cause a significant response that leads to cell death by apoptosis. This type of direct synergy may also considerably increase the therapeutic response to a given anticancer treatment. Work in our own laboratory has shown that the addition of curcumin and EGCG to cancerous cells subjected to weak doses of radiation causes a spectacular increase in the response of these cells to treatment (**see Figure 35, below**).

Synergy is also often involved in indirect mechanisms. The foods that we eat on a daily basis contain a host of molecules without any anticancer activity *per se*, but which can nevertheless have a considerable impact on cancer prevention by increasing the quantity (and thus the potential anticancer activity) of

EXAMPLES OF DIRECT SYNERGY

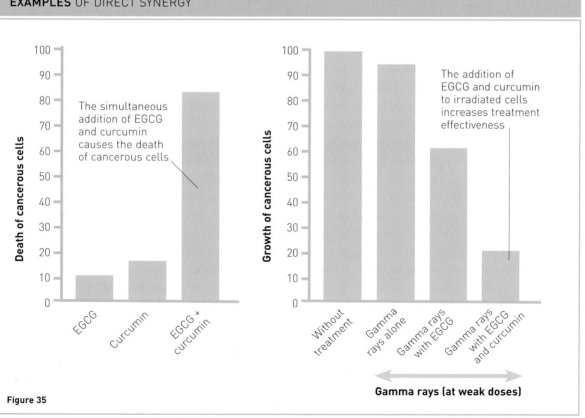

The simultaneous addition of EGCG and curcumin causes the death of cancerous cells

The addition of EGCG and curcumin to irradiated cells increases treatment effectiveness

Gamma rays (at weak doses)

Figure 35

another anticancer molecule in the bloodstream, by slowing down its elimination, or by increasing its absorption (**see Figure 34, p.176**).

One of the best examples of this indirect synergy is the action of piperine, a molecule that is present in pepper. Piperine increases by a factor of 1,000 the absorption of curcumin (**see Figure 36, below**); the presence of piperine allows the amount of curcumin present in the body to achieve levels sufficient to modify the aggressive behavior of cancerous cells. In our opinion, not only does this synergy illustrate the necessity of adopting a diverse diet to maximize possible health benefits, it also makes the substitution of supplements containing isolated molecules for these precious whole foods an inconsistent and ultimately unwise choice (**see Chapter 17, p.165**).

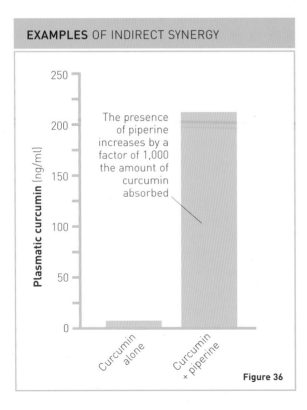

EXAMPLES OF INDIRECT SYNERGY

Plasmatic curcumin (ng/ml)

The presence of piperine increases by a factor of 1,000 the amount of curcumin absorbed

Curcumin alone

Curcumin + piperine

Figure 36

A DIET TO HELP PREVENT CANCER

The diet we recommend should be taken as a guide to a carefully outlined program for health whose every ingredient, without exception, possesses anticancer properties. In other words, this is a diet in which each and every component supplies the organism with a daily dose of the ammunition needed to fight the development of cancer. If the diet seems at first somewhat severe, this is because it was designed for high-risk patients, such as those who have already fought the disease and are in remission, so that they might be given every possible chance to prevent the disease's recurrence.

Indeed, the food guide that we propose can be particularly useful for persons at high risk for developing cancer, whether because of their family history or because they have already been afflicted by the disease. This type of prevention, known as secondary prevention, is different from the primary prevention we just described, in which the regular consumption of foods rich in anticancer compounds curbs the development of cancer by attacking it from the point of its emergence. In secondary prevention, these foods induce an important biological response in patients, acting to limit as much as possible the development of tumoral foci that may not have been completely eliminated by conventional surgery, radiotherapy, or chemotherapy treatment.

Don't wait until it's too late

However, our recommendations may be applied in their entirety by any person wishing to reduce his or her risk of developing cancer. We have observed the basic principle throughout this book: certain foods constitute exceptional sources of anticancer molecules, and the simple fact of adding them to your daily diet may have an extraordinary impact on the incidence of the principal cancers currently plaguing our society. Incorporating cruciferous vegetables, garlic and its cousins, soy, and certain fruits into your diet as much as possible will supply your body with levels of anticancer molecules that are impossible to attain with other vegetables. Let us also reemphasize the central role played by soy, green tea, and turmeric in the difference between the cancer rates experienced by East and West – these foods are undoubtedly major allies in cancer prevention.

Advocating the preferential consumption of the foods described here does not mean that other foods, such as beans, artichokes, eggplant, bell peppers, mushrooms, apples, bananas, and other delicious fruits and vegetables just as essential to a diverse diet are not worth eating! On the contrary – given the troubling overall state of diet in the West, any change in dietary habits that is characterized by the increased consumption of fruits and vegetables is very positive and should be encouraged.

Five a day is the minimum
Despite many years of intensive publicity campaigns and government programs designed to promote the increased consumption of fruits and vegetables, barely one-quarter of the population currently respects the minimum recommended amount of about five daily servings of these foods. Indeed, the consumption of fruits and vegetables is actually decreasing in certain areas of the globe. This disturbing situation can be blamed on several factors, notably a certain number of tenacious myths that seem to dampen the enthusiasm of consumers toward products of plant origin (**see box, p.181**). Given the essential role of fruits and vegetables in an overall cancer prevention strategy, it goes without saying that changing negative preconceptions toward these foods is an important prerequisite to any significant reduction in the cancer levels now afflicting us.

Other foods you should include
The choice of fruits and vegetables included in our recommended diet is based on currently available knowledge as to the anticancer potential of these foods. However, research being a dynamic process, it is possible and even very likely that other anticancer molecules will be identified in the next few years, and these new discoveries will prompt us to improve on the diet by making it even more diverse.

We already know that many other foods apart from the foods discussed in this book also contain important quantities of phytochemical compounds, and that these other compounds have all been suggested as having in varying degrees the potential to interfere with the processes involved in the development of cancer (**see Table 22, p.180**). We can cite as an example the pigments and complex sugars present in certain marine algae (wakame, hijiki, and arame) eaten daily by the Japanese, which may prevent the development of certain cancers, especially breast cancer. It is equally fascinating to observe that many herbs and spices used as seasonings contain large quantities of molecules that act as anti-inflammatory compounds, which also reduce the risks of developing certain chronic diseases such as cancer.

Ginger is the best example of this latter category. One of the principal molecules present in this spicy root, known as gingerol, has often been put forward as a powerful potential anticancer agent, for its anti-inflammatory properties as well as its inhibiting activity on cancerous cells.

OTHER FOOD (DIETARY) SOURCES RICH IN **ANTICANCER PHYTOCHEMICAL COMPOUNDS**	
Food	**Phytochemical compound**
Alfalfa sprouts	Coumestrol
Apple	Quercetin
Artichoke	Silymarin
Avocado	Alpha-carotene
Barley	Phytates
Basil and rosemary	Ursolic acid
Bok choy	Dithiolthione
Black tea	Theaflavin
Capers	Kampferol
Celery	Apigenin
Cherries	Cyanidin
Chili pepper	Capsaicin
Clove	Eugenol
Eggplant	Nasuin
Fennel, anis, coriander	Anethol
Ginger	6-gingerol
Grapefruit	Naringenin
Lentils	Lignans
Lettuce	Zeaxanthin
Mangoes	Beta-cryptoxanthin
Marine algae	Fucoxanthins
Parsley	Apigenin
Pear	Hydroxycinnamic acid
Shiitake mushrooms	Lentinan
Spinach	Lutein
Thyme	Luteolin
Wheat bran	Fiber

Table 22

We should also mention that herbs such as parsley, thyme, mint, and capers contain extraordinary quantities of the polyphenols apigenin, luteolin, and kampferol. These molecules exhibit important inhibitory activity on the growth of cancerous cells as well as behavior that seems to prevent the development of tumors in laboratory animals. It is becoming more and more apparent that seasoning a dish is not just a detail in culinary art, but may also be an essential feature in cancer prevention.

THE IMPORTANCE OF EATING HEALTHILY AND WITH PLEASURE

It goes without saying: in order to fully avail yourself of the benefits of the foods we have described, it is important to seek out the many sources of recipes that use these ingredients in the preparation of simple and delicious meals. Preventing cancer through diet has the potential to become a very pleasant exercise, if we prepare food with an eye toward creating a genuine feast!

We recommend going about this in a very simple way: by purchasing several cookbooks that showcase the cuisines of the principal culinary traditions discussed in this book. There is no point in reinventing the wheel, as it were. The inhabitants of the Middle East have been consuming legumes in various ways for at least 3,000 years and have acquired considerable know-how in the preparation of dishes based on these vegetables. Asian cuisines offer multiple possibilities for using soy in all its forms, and cookbooks can instruct you in the best ways of reclaiming this food for yourself, as well as

NEGATIVE MYTHS SURROUNDING FRUITS AND VEGETABLES

Myth 1. Fruits and vegetables contain pesticide residues that cause cancer.

False. Pesticide residues in fruits and vegetables are present in trace amounts and no study has ever established a link between these residues and cancer. The opposite is true: the consumption of fruits and vegetables has constantly been linked to a decrease in the risk of developing cancer, and there is no doubt that the benefits associated with an increased intake of these foods exceed many times over any hypothetical negative effects that trace amounts of contaminants might cause. A simple way of eliminating virtually all of these residues is to rinse fruits and vegetables thoroughly with water; you may also choose to purchase fruits and vegetables grown without pesticides.

Myth 2. Fruits and vegetables are the result of genetic manipulation, and genetically modified organisms (GMOs) are harmful to health.

False. The great majority of fruits and vegetables currently available come from varieties that are the product of natural selection. No foreign genetic material has ever been introduced into these foods, and they may be considered entirely natural. As for the fruits and vegetables that have been genetically modified, no study has succeeded in establishing any carcinogenic character in these foods. These results are unsurprising, given that the proteins created during genetic manipulation are destroyed in digestion and thus cannot have any real impact on nutritional intake. The real problem with GMOs is environmental. Its most important aspect concerns the extremely negative impact of GMOs on the diversity of living plant species. This is a serious problem and we share the concerns of those who oppose GMOs on this count. In our opinion, it is imperative that the efforts now deployed in the production of genetically modified organisms be limited to a strict minimum in order to avoid a potential ecological catastrophe.

Myth 3. Only organic fruits and vegetables offer real health benefits.

False. Every study that succeeded in establishing the anticancer potential of fruits and vegetables focused on the consumption of foods cultivated in "traditional" ways. Eating foods labeled "organic" is not a prerequisite for benefiting from these foods. Even though the pesticide-free cultivation of plants may stimulate the plants' defense systems, allowing them to produce slightly higher quantities of anticancer phytochemical compounds, it is misleading to think that only organic fruits and vegetables can have a positive impact on health. In fact, it would be better to consume many "standard" fruits and vegetables on a daily basis than to only occasionally eat organic foods, if the generally higher cost of organically grown produce is what is preventing you from regularly buying fruits and vegetables.

experimenting with other healthful vegetables often used in these cuisines, especially different types of cabbage.

Both Mediterranean and Japanese cuisines have raised the preparation of fish and seafood to the level of an art form, and they are an indispensable reference for guiding you in the planning of meals based around these foods. The same goes for the tomato in Italian and Spanish cooking, or the different curries widespread in Indian cuisine.

These recipes provide a golden opportunity to prepare delicious, flavorful meals inspired by the principles that we have elaborated throughout this book. "Delicious" is the key word here, since eating in a healthy manner requires first and foremost the ability to take real pleasure in eating. For most people, a diet is the height of boredom, synonymous with punishment and deprivation. On the contrary! The program we recommend, far from being a kind of punishment, should be seen as its own reward! Enjoying access to the thousands of recipes that make use of tasty, healthy ingredients and constantly varying menus and meals in order to include many of the hundreds of fruits and vegetables now available is much more about being an epicure than an exercise in austerity.

IN CONCLUSION

Choosing to modify your diet in order to include certain foods that are exceptional sources of anticancer molecules represents one of the best weapons currently at our disposal in the fight against cancer.

There is nothing extravagant or revolutionary about these changes. This is about reemphasizing the important role of diet in daily life by paying greater attention to the impact of the foods we eat on general wellbeing. We are convinced that you will take enormous satisfaction in implementing these modifications, whether for the pure gastronomic pleasure of it, or for the feeling of satisfaction in actively building up your body's defense systems by supplying them with a daily dose of these medicines of dietary origin.

We are immensely privileged to have access to abundant food resources. Using these resources not only as necessary nourishment but also as substances that can reduce the incidence of serious disease may represent one of the most significant advances in our fight against cancer. Diet is at the heart of human civilization. It is an expression of humanity's ingenuity in exploring its environment in order to discover new foods, and an illustration of its constant quest for wellbeing. It is impossible to accept that a mere century's worth of industrialization of food and agriculture has succeeded in destroying this heritage, in denying a certain collective wisdom, and in laying waste to its basic principles.

Preventing cancer through diet is first and foremost about finding and reclaiming the essence of the ancient dietary traditions elaborated and developed over millennia by human civilizations. It is about paying homage to the inestimable knowledge gathered by thousands of generations of women who needed to provide their children with the foods necessary for good health, while seeking the best ways to prepare these foods so that eating them would become a joyfully shared experience. It is about showing respect to the most formidable experiment ever undertaken by humanity, without which we would not exist. Put very simply, preventing cancer through diet is about renewing our ties with the very essence of the human condition.

chocolate

avocado

broccoli

tea

Bibliography

Chapter 1
To learn more about...
... the principles at the heart of a healthy diet:
- A. Weil. Eating Well for Optimum Health: The Essential Guide to Food, Diet, and Nutrition. Knopf, 2000, 320 pages.

... the damage caused by obesity:
- E. E. Calle, R. Kaaks. Overweight, obesity and cancer: epidemiological evidence and proposed mechanisms. Nature Reviews on Cancer, 2004; 4: 579-591.
- S.J. Olshansky, Douglas J. Passaro, Ronald C. Hershow et al. A potential decline in life expectancy in the United States in the 21st century. N. Eng. J. Med. 2005; 352: 1138-1144.

... the impact of diet on cancer:
- R. Doll, R.Peto. The causes of cancer: quantitative estimates of avoidable risks of cancer in the United States today. J. Natl. Cancer Inst. 1981; 66: 1196-1265.
- World Cancer Research Fund/American Institute for Cancer Research. Food, Nutrition and the Prevention of Cancer. A Global Perspective. 1997, 670 pages.
- D. Heber, G.L. Blackburn, V. L. W. Go (Editors). Nutritional Oncology. Academic Press, 1999, 632 pages.
- T. J. Key, N.E. Allen, E.A. Spencer, R.C. Travis. The effect of diet on risk of cancer. Lancet 2002; 360: 861-868.

Chapter 2
To learn more about...
... the appearance of cancer:
- Les sociétés cellulaires. Dossier Pour la Science No. 19, April 1998.
- W. Gibbs. L'imbroglio génétique du cancer. Pour la Science 2003; 310 pages.
- M. H. Goyns. Cancer and You. How to

Stack the Odds in Your Favor. Harwood Academic Publishers, 1999, 159 pages.
- D. Hanahan, R. A. Weinberg. The hallmarks of cancer. Cell 2000; 100: 57-70.

Chapter 3
To learn more about...
... the treatment of cancer:
- J. F. Bishop, Ed. Cancer Facts. A Concise Oncology Text. Harwood Academic Publishers, 1999, 411 pages.

... angiogenesis and the angiogenic effect of elements of diet:
- J. Folkman. Angiogenesis in cancer, vascular, rheumatoid and other diseases. Nature Med. 1995; 1: 27-31.
- F. Tosetti, N. Ferrari, S. de Flora,a A. Albini. "Angioprevention": angiogenesis is a common and key target for cancer chemopreventive agents. FASEB J. 2002; 16: 2-14.

... metronomic therapy:
- R.S. Kerbel, B.A. Kamen. The anti-angiogenic basis of metronomic chemotherapy. Nature Reviews on Cancer 2004; 4: 423-436.

Chapter 4
To learn more about...
... the history of cancer treatment:
- S.I. Hajdu. Greco-Roman thought about cancer. Cancer 2004; 100: 2048-2051.
- I.M. Lonie, Hippocrates, E.T. Withington, G.E.R. Lloyd, J. Chadwick, W.N. Mann. Hippocratic Writings. Penguin Classics, 1984, 384 pages.

... tumoral microfoci:
- W.C. Black, H.G. Welch. Advances in diagnostic imaging and overestimation

of disease prevalence and the benefits of therapy. N. Eng. J. Med. 1993; 328: 1237-1243.
- J. Folkman, R. Kalluri. Cancer without disease. Nature 2004; 427: 787.

... the prevention of cancer through diet:
- A. Gescher, U. Pastorino, S.M. Plummer, M.M. Manson. Suppression of tumour development by substances derived from the diet: mechanisms and clinical implications. Br. J. Clin. Pharmacol. 1998; 45: 1-12.
- M.L. McCullough, E.L. Giovannucci. Diet and cancer prevention. Oncogene 2004; 23: 6349-6364.

Chapter 5
To learn more about...
... phytochemical compounds:
- Y.-J. Surh. Cancer chemoprevention with dietary phytochemicals. Nature Reviews on Cancer 2003; 3: 768-780.
- T. Dorai, B.B. Aggarwal. Role of chemopreventive agents in cancer therapy. Cancer Lett. 2004; 215: 129-140.
- C. Manach, A. Scalbert, C. Morand, C. Rémésy, L. Jiménez. Polyphenols: food sources and bioavailability. Am. J. Clin. Nutr. 2004; 79: 727-747.
- A.M. Bode, Z. Dong. Targeting signal transduction pathways by chemopreventive agents. Mut. Res. 2004; 555: 33-51.

... vitamin supplements and cancer:
- The ATBC Study Group. The effect of vitamin E and beta-carotene on the incidence of lung cancer and other cancers in male smokers. N. Engl. J. Med. 1994; 330: 1029-1035.
- E.R. Miller, R. Pastor-Barriuso, D. Dalal,

R.A. Riemersma, L.J. Appel, E. Guallar. Meta-analysis: High-dosage vitamin E supplementation may increase all-cause mortality. Ann. Intern. Med. 2005; 142: 37-46.

Chapter 6
To learn more about...
... cancer prevention with cruciferous vegetables:

● D.T.H. Verhoeven, R.A. Goldbohm, G. van Poppel, H. Verhagen, P.A. van den Brandt. Epidemiological studies on Brassica vegetables and cancer risk. Cancer Epidemiol. Biomarkers Prev. 1996; 5: 733-748.

● P. Talalay, J.W. Fahey. Phytochemicals from cruciferous plants protect against cancer by modulating carcinogen metabolism. J. Nutr. 2001; 131: 3027S-3033S.

● Y.-S. Keum, W.-S. Jeong, A.N. T. Kong. Chemoprevention by isothiocyanates and their underlying molecular signaling mechanisms. Mut. Res. 2004; 555: 191-202.

● S.J. London, J.-M. Yuan, F.-L. Chung, Y.-T. Gao, G.A. Coetzee, R.K. Ross, M.C. Yu. Isothiocyanates, glutathione S-transferase M1 and T1 polymorphisms, and lung-cancer risk: a prospective study of men in Shanghai, China. Lancet 2000; 356: 724-729.

... glucosinolates in general:

● G.R. Fenwick, R.K. Heaney, W.J. Mullin. Glucosinolates and their breakdown products in food and food plants. CRC Critical Rev. Food Sci. and Nutr. 1983; 18: 123-201.

● H.L. Bradlow, D.W. Sepkovic, N.T. Telang, M.P. Osborne. Multifunctional aspects of the action of Indole-3-carbinol as an antitumor agent. Ann. N.Y. Acad. Sci. 1999; 889: 204-213.

... sulforaphane:

● **Y. Zhang, P. Talalay, C.G. Cho, G.H. Posner. A major inducer of anticarcinogenic protective enzymes from broccoli: isolation and elucidation of structure. Proc. Natl. Acad. Sci. USA 1992; 89: 2399-2403.

● J.W. Fahey, Y. Zhang, P. Talalay. Broccoli sprouts: an exceptionally rich source of inducers of enzymes that protect against chemical carcinogens. Proc. Natl. Acad. Sci. USA 1997; 94: 10367-10372.

● J.W. Fahey, X. Haristoy, P.M. Dolan, T.W. Kensler, I. Scholtus, K.K. Stephenson, P. Talalay, A. Lozniewski. Sulforaphane inhibits extracellular, intracellular and antibiotic-resistant strains of Helicobacter pylori and prevents benzo[a]pyrene-induces stomach tumors. Proc. Natl. Acad. Sci. USA 2002; 99: 7610-7615.

● D. Gingras, M. Gendron, D. Boivin, A. Moghrabi, Y. Théôret, R. Béliveau. Induction of medulloblastoma cell apoptosis by sulforaphane, a dietary anticarcinogen from Brassica vegetables. Cancer Lett. 2004; 203: 35-43.

Chapter 7
To learn more about...
... the anticancer effects of vegetables from the Allium family:

● A.W. Hsing, A.P. Chokkalingam, Y.T. Gao, M.P. Madigan, J. Deng, G. Gridley, J.F. Fraumeni. Allium vegetables and risk of prostate cancer: a population-based study. J. Natl. Cancer Inst. 2002; 94: 1648-1651.

● A.T. Fleischauer, L. Arab. Garlic and cancer: a critical review of the epidemiologic literature. J Nutr. 2001; 131: 1032S-1040S.

● A. Herman-Antosiewicz, S.V. Singh. Signal transduction pathways leading to cell cycle arrest and apoptosis induction in cancer cells by Allium vegetable-derived organosulfur compounds: a review. Mut. Res. 2004; 555: 121-131.

● M. Demeule, M. Brossard, S. Turcotte, A. Régina, R. Jodoin, R. Béliveau. Diallyl disulfide, a chemopreventive agent in garlic, induces multidrug resistance-associated protein 2 expression. Biochem. Biophys. Res. Commun. 2004; 324: 937-945.

... the chemical composition of garlic and onions:

● E. Block. The chemistry of garlic and onion. Sci. Am. 1985; 252: 114-119.

Chapter 8
To learn more about...
... hormone-dependent cancers:

● M. Clemons, P. Goss. Estrogen and the risk of breast cancer. N. Eng. J. Med. 2001; 344: 276-285.

... the biological properties of isoflavones:

● P.J. Magee, I.R. Rowland. Phyto-oestrogens, their mechanism of action: current evidence for a role in breast and prostate cancer. Br. J. Nutrition 2004; 91: 513-531.

● F.H. Sarkar, Y. Li. Mechanisms of cancer chemoprevention by soy isoflavone genistein. Cancer Metast. Rev. 2002; 21: 265-280.

● T. Akiyama, J. Ishida, S. Nakagawa, H. Ogawara, S.-I. Watanabe, N. Itoh, M. Shibuya, Y. Fukami. Genistein, a specific inhibitor of tyrosine-specific protein kinases. J. Biol. Chem. 1987; 262: 5592-5595.

... the impact of soy and isoflavones on the development of cancer:

● H. Adlercreutz. Phyto-oestrogens and cancer. Lancet Oncol. 2002; 3: 364-373.

● S. Yamamoto, T. Sobue, M. Kobayashi, S. Sasaki, S. Tsugane. Soy, isoflavones, and breast cancer risk in Japan. J. Natl. Cancer Inst. 2003; 95: 906-913.

● A.H. Wu, P. Wan, J. Hankin, C.-C. Tseng, M.C. Yu, M.C. Pike. Adolescent and adult soy intake and risk of breast cancer in Asian-Americans. Carcinogenesis 2002; 23: 1491-1496.

● M.M. Lee, S.L. Gomez, J.S. Chang, M. Wey R.-T. Wang, A.W. Hsing. Soy and isoflavone consumption in relation to prostate cancer risk in China. Cancer Epidemiol. Biomarkers Prev. 2003; 12: 665-668.

● M.J. Messina, C.L. Loprinzi. Soy for

breast cancer survivors: a critical review of the literature. J. Nutr. 2001; 131: 3095S-3108S.

• C.D. Allred, K.F. Allred, Y.H. Ju, T.S. Goeppinger, D.R. Doerge, W.G. Helferich. Soy processing influences growth of estrogen-dependent breast cancer tumors. Carcinogenesis 2004; 25: 1649-1657.

Chapter 9
To learn more about…
… turmeric and curcumin:

• B.B. Aggarwal, A. Kumar, M.S. Aggarwal, S. Shishodia. Curcumin derived from turmeric (Curcuma longa): A spice for all seasons. In Phytochemicals in Cancer Chemoprevention, D. Bagchi, H.G. Preuss, Eds., 1-24.

Chapter 10
To learn more about…
… green tea:

• L.A. Mitscher, V. Dolby, The Green Tea Book. China's Fountain of Youth, Avery, 1998, 186 pages.

• D. Rosen, The Book of Green Tea, Storey Publishing, 1998, 160 pages.

… the anticancer properties of green tea:

• C.S. Yang, Z.Y. Wang. Tea and cancer. J. Natl. Cancer Inst. 1993; 85, 1038-1049.

• V. Crespy, G. Williamson. A review of the health effects of green tea catechins in in vivo animal models. J. Nutr. 2004; 134: 3431S-3440S.

• R. Béliveau, D. Gingras. Green tea: prevention and treatment of cancer by nutraceuticals. Lancet 2004; 364: 1021-1022.

• M. Demeule, J. Michaud-Lévesque, B. Annabi, D. Gingras, D. Boivin, J. Jodoin, S. Lamy, Y. Bertrand, R. Béliveau. Green tea catechins as novel antitumor and antiangiogenic compounds. Curr. Med. Chem. Anti-Canc. Agents. 2002; 2: 441-63.

… the principal anticancer compound in green tea, EGCG:

• Y. Cao. R. Cao. Angiogenesis inhibited by drinking tea. Nature 1999; 398: 381.

• S. Lamy, D. Gingras, R. Béliveau. Green tea catechins inhibit vascular endothelial growth factor receptor phosphorylation. Cancer Res. 2002; 62: 381-385.

• B. Annabi, Y.T. Lee, C. Martel, A. Pilorget, J.P. Bahary, R. Béliveau. Radiation induced-tubulogenesis in endothelial cells is antagonized by the antiangiogenic properties of green tea polyphenol (-) epigallocatechin-3-gallate. Cancer Biol. Ther. 2003; 2: 642-649.

• A. Pilorget, V. Berthet, J. Luis, A. Moghrabi, B. Annabi, R. Béliveau. Medulloblastoma cell invasion is inhibited by green tea (-)epigallocatechin-3-gallate. J. Cell. Biochem. 2003; 90: 745-755.

• J. Jodoin, M. Demeule, R. Béliveau. Inhibition of the multidrug resistance P-glycoprotein activity by green tea polyphenols. Biochim. Biophys. Acta. 2002; 1542: 149-159.

• M. Demeule, M. Brossard, M. Pagé, D. Gingras, R. Béliveau. Matrix metalloproteinase inhibition by green tea catechins. Biochim. Biophys. Acta. 2000; 1478: 51-60.

Chapter 11
To learn more about…
… the anticancer effects of strawberries, raspberries, and ellagic acid:

• S.M. Hannum. Potential impact of strawberries on human health: a review of the science. Crit. Rev. Food Sci. Nutr. 2004; 44: 1-17.

• L.A. Kresty, M.A. Morse, C. Morgan, P.S. Carlton, J. Lu, A. Gupta, M. Blackwood, G. D. Stoner. Chemoprevention of esophageal tumorigenesis by dietary administration of lyophilized black raspberries. Cancer Res. 2001; 61: 6112-6119.

• P.S. Carlton, L.A. Kresty, J.C. Siglin, M.A. Morse, J. Lu, C. Morgan, G.D. Stoner. Inhibition of N-nitrosomethylbenzylamine-induced tumorigenesis in the rat esophagus by dietary freeze-dried strawberries. Carcinogenesis 2001; 22: 441-446.

• L. Labrecque, S. Lamy, A. Chapus, S. Mihoubi, Y. Durocher, B. Cass, M.W. Bojanowski, D. Gingras, R. Béliveau. Combined inhibition of PDGF and VEGF receptors by ellagic acid, a dietary-derived phenolic compound. Carcinogenesis 2005; 26: 821-826.

… the anticancer potential of blueberries and the anthocyanidins:

• J.M. Kong, L.S. Chia, N.-K. Goh, T.-F. Chia, R. Brouillard. Analysis and biological activities of anthocyanins. Phytochemistry 2003; 64: 923-933.

• S. Lamy, M. Blanchette, J. Michaud-Lévesque, R. Lafleur, Y. Durocher, A. Moghrabi, D. Gingras, R. Béliveau (2005) Delphinidin, a dietary anthocyanidin, inhibits VEGFR-2 activity and in vitro angiogenesis (in preparation).

… the proanthocyanidins and their importance:

• S.E. Rasmussen, H. Frederiksen, K.S. Krogholm, L. Poulsen. Dietary proanthocyanidins: Occurrence, dietary intake, bioavailability, and protection against cardiovascular disease. Mol. Nutr. Food Res. 2005; 49: 159-174.

Chapter 12
To learn more about…
… the impact of omega-3s on cardiovascular diseases:

• P.M. Kris-Etherton, W.S. Harris, L.J. Appel. Fish consumption, fish oil, omega-3 fatty acids, and cardiovascular disease. Circulation 2002; 106: 2747.

… the impact of omega-3s on cancer prevention:

• D.P. Rose, J.M. Connolly. Omega-3 fatty acids as cancer chemopreventive agents. Pharm. Ther. 1999; 83: 217-244.

• S.C. Larsson, M. Kumlin, M. Ingelman-Sundberg, A. Wolk. Dietary long-chain n-3 fatty acids for the prevention of cancer: a review of potential mechanisms. Am. J. Clin. Nutr. 2004; 79: 935-945.

Chapter 13
To learn more about…
… the anticancer potential of tomatoes:

● E. Giovannucci. A review of epidemiologic studies of tomatoes, lycopene, and prostate cancer. Exp. Biol. Med. 2002; 227: 852-859.

● J.K. Campbell, K. Canene-Adams, B.L. Lindshield, T.W.-M. Boileau, S.K. Clinton, J. W. Erdman. Tomato phytochemicals and prostate cancer risk. J. Nutr. 2004; 134: 3486S-3492S.

● K. Wertz, U. Siler, R. Goralczyk. Lycopene: modes of action to promote prostate health. Arch. Biochem. Biophys. 2004; 430: 127-134.

Chapter 14
To learn more about…
… the ancient therapeutic uses of citrus fruits:

● B.A. Arias, L. Ramon-Laca. Pharmacological properties of citrus and their ancient and medieval uses in the Mediterranean region. J. Ethnopharm. 2005; 97: 89-95.

… the anticancer potential of citrus fruits:

● J.A. Manthey, N. Guthrie, K. Grohmann. Biological properties of citrus flavonoids pertaining to cancer and inflammation. Curr. Med. Chem. 2001; 8: 135-153.

● P.L. Crowell. Prevention and therapy of cancer by dietary monoterpenes. J. Nutr. 1999; 129: 775S-778S.

Chapter 15
To learn more about…
… the impact of red wine on cardiovascular diseases:

● A.S. St-Leger, A.L. Cochrane, F. Moore. Factors associated with cardiac mortality in developed countries with particular reference to the consumption of wine. Lancet 1979; 1: 1017-1020.

● S. Renaud, M. de Lorgeril. Wine, alcohol, platelets, and the French paradox for coronary heart disease. Lancet 1992; 339: 1523-1526.

● J.B. German, R.L. Walzem. The health benefits of wine. Annu. Rev. Nutr. 2000; 20: 561-593.

● A. Di Castelnuovo, S. Rotondo, L. Iacoviello, M.B. Donati, G. de Gateno. Meta-analysis of wine and beer consumption in relation to vascular risk. Circulation 2002; 105: 2836-2844.

… the impact of red wine on the development of cancer:

● M. Gronbaek, U. Becker, D. Johansen, A. Gottschau, P. Schnohr, H.O. Hein, G. Jensen, T.I. Sorensen . Type of alcohol consumed and mortality from all causes, coronary heart disease, and cancer. Ann. Intern. Med. 2000; 133: 411-419.

…resveratrol:

● M. Jang, L. Cai, G.O. Udeani, K.V. Slowing, C.F. Thomas et al. Cancer chemopreventive activity of resveratrol, a natural product derived from grapes. Science 1997; 275: 218-220.

● J.G. Wood, B. Rogina, S. Lavu, K. Howitz, S.L. Helfand, M. Tatar, D. Sinclair. Sirtuin activators mimic caloric restriction and delay ageing in metazoans. Nature 2004; 430: 686-689.

Chapter 16
To learn more about…
… the ancient uses of cacao:

● T.L. Dillinger, P. Barriga, S. Escarcega, M. Jimenez, D.S. Lowe, L.E. Grivetti. Food of the gods: cure for humanity? A cultural history of the medicinal and ritual use of chocolate. J. Nutr. 2000; 130: 2057S-2072S

● W.J. Hurst, S.M. Tarka, T.G. Powis, F. Valdez, T.R. Hester. Cacao usage by the earliest Maya civilization. Nature 2002; 418: 289-290.

… the beneficial properties of cacao:

● J.H. Weisburger. Chemopreventive effects of cocoa polyphenols on chronic diseases. Exp. Biol. Med. 2001; 226:, 891-897.

● C.L. Keen, R.R. Holt, P.I. Oteiza, C.G. Fraga, H.H. Schmitz. Cocoa antioxidants and cardiovascular health. Am. J. Clin. Nutr. 2005; 81: 298S-303S.

● T.P. Kenny, C.L. Keen, P. Jones, H.-J. Kung, H.H. Schmitz, M.E. Gershwin. Pentameric procyanidins isolated from Theobroma cacao seeds selectively downregulate ErbB2 in human aortic endothelial cells. Exp. Biol. Med. 2004; 229: 255-263.

Index

Acknowledgments

Authors' acknowledgments

Our thanks go first to all children suffering from cancer and their families, whose courage inspired the writing of this book. Thank you to the Charles Bruneau Foundation, whose encouragement and financial support allowed us to develop the nutratherapy program. Thank you to the UQAM Foundation, which supported us by endowing the Chair in Cancer Prevention and Treatment. Thank you to Dr. Judah Folkman, whose visionary ideas on cancer treatment served as the starting point for the principles discussed in this book. Thank you to Dr. Jean-Marie Leclerc, without whom none of this would have been possible, for his generous energy and the clarity of his vision. Thank you to Dr. Mark Bernstein, head of the Hemato-Oncology Division at the CHU Sainte-Justine Research Center, for his support in this transitional research approach. Thank you to our colleagues at the Hemato-Oncology Division at the CHU Sainte-Justine Research Center for their incredible devotion in the fight against cancer, and for their dynamic response to new research ideas. Thank you to all the members of the division – nurses, pharmacists, volunteers, therapists – for their immense commitment and their generous involvement in the lives of young cancer patients. Thank you to Dr. Lise Tremblay for her judicious comments on the early versions of the manuscript and her support in all the subsequent stages of the writing and preparation of this book. Thank you to Line Larivière for her suggestions and to Yumeji Asaoka for the French translation of the passage from Kissa Yôjôki. Thank you to Dr. Hélène Rousseau for her critical reading and her constant encouragement. Thank you to Dr. Sylvie Lamy for her perseverance, her perfectionist's work, and her unshakeable faith in our research. Thank you to all of our student research assistants in the Molecular Medicine Laboratory, whose research work led to the first discoveries in nutratherapy, for their extraordinary enthusiasm in advancing human knowledge. Thank you to Professor Ben Sulsky for guiding us in the first stages of this approach, for his unwavering friendship, his faith in science, and his very great compassion toward suffering humanity.

Publisher's acknowledgments

Dorling Kindersley would like to thank senior editor Jill Hamilton for her help in producing this book; Alyson Silverwood for proofreading; and Lynn Bresler for the index. Thank you to Lisa Hark, PhD RD, for reviewing the US edition, to Darwin Deen, MD, and to Lyndel Costain, B.Sc.RD, for reviewing the UK edition. Originally published as *Les Aliments Contre le Cancer*, Éditions du Trécarré, 2005; original design concept by Cyclone Design Communications; English translation by Milena Stojanac.